Your Best Face

OTHER HAY HOUSE TITLES OF RELATED INTEREST

Books

*The Body "Knows": How to Tune In to Your Body and Improve
Your Health,* by Caroline M. Sutherland, Medical Intuitive

Growing Older, Growing Better, by Amy E. Dean

*Love Your Body: A Positive Affirmation Guide for Loving
and Appreciating Your Body,* by Louise L. Hay

Ultimate Pilates: Achieve the Perfect Body Shape, by Dreas Reyneke

*Your Personality, Your Health: Connecting Personality with the Human
Energy System, Chakras, and Wellness,* by Carol Ritberger, Ph.D.

Audio Programs

Awakening the Goddesses Within, A Dialogue Between
Agapi Stassinopoulos and Deepak Chopra, M.D.

*Healing Meditations: Enhance Your Immune System
and Find the Key to Good Health,* by Bernie Siegel, M.D.

Live Long and Feel Good, by Andrew Weil, M.D., with Michael Toms

*Women's Bodies, Women's Choices: Creating Physical and Emotional
Health and Healing,* by Christiane Northrup, M.D.

Card Decks

Healthy Body Cards, by Louise L. Hay

OM Yoga Flash Cards, by Cyndi Lee

Self-Care Cards, by Cheryl Richardson

All of the above are available at your local bookstore,
or may be ordered through Hay House, Inc.:

(800) 654-5126 or **(760) 431-7695**
(800) 650-5115 (fax) or **(760) 431-6948 (fax)**
www.hayhouse.com

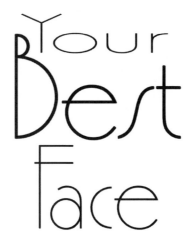

Your Best Face

Looking Your Best Without Plastic Surgery

Brandith Irwin, M.D.,
and Mark McPherson, Ph.D.

Hay House, Inc.
Carlsbad, California • Sydney, Australia
Canada • Hong Kong • United Kingdom

Published and distributed in the United States by: Hay House, Inc.,
P.O. Box 5100, Carlsbad, CA 92018-5100 • (800) 654-5126 • (800) 650-5115 (fax)
www.hayhouse.com • *Published and distributed in Australia by:* Hay House
Australia Pty Ltd, P.O. Box 515, Brighton-Le-Sands, NSW 2216 • *phone:* 1800 023 516
e-mail: info@hayhouse.com.au • *Distributed in the United Kingdom by:*
Airlift, 8 The Arena, Mollison Ave., Enfield, Middlesex, United Kingdom EN3 7NL
Distributed in Canada by: Raincoast, 9050 Shaughnessy St., Vancouver, B.C.,
Canada V6P 6E5

Editorial supervision: Jill Kramer • *Design:* Jenn Ramsey • *Index:* Debra Graf

The authors of this book do not dispense medical advice or prescribe the use of any technique as a form of treatment for physical or medical problems without the advice of a physician, either directly or indirectly. The intent of the authors is only to offer information of a general nature to help you in your quest for emotional and spiritual well-being. In the event you use any of the information in this book for yourself, which is your constitutional right, the authors and the publisher assume no responsibility for your actions.

Library of Congress Cataloging-in-Publication Data

Irwin, Brandith.
  Your best face : looking your best without plastic surgery / Brandith Irwin and
Mark McPherson.
      p. cm.
    Includes index.
    ISBN 1-56170-953-0
    1. Skin—Care and hygiene. 2. Beauty, Personal. 3. Skin—Laser surgery.
  4. Surgery, Plastic. I. McPherson, Mark, 1955- II. Title.
    RL87 .I794 2002
    646.7'26—dc21

                                            2002005198

                          ISBN 1-56170-953-0

                    05 04 03 02   4 3 2 1
                    1st printing, October 2002

            Printed in the United States of America

This book is dedicated to my patients,
whose excellent questions inspired it.

CONTENTS

Part I: WRINKLES

Chapter 1:
Fine Wrinkles

WHAT ARE THE POSSIBLE CAUSES?
Sun Damage • Dry Conditions • Weather • Irritation from Products

WHAT ARE THE POSSIBLE TREATMENTS?
Moisterizers • Laser Photorejuvenation • Microdermabrasion •
Gycolic and "Chemical" Peels

Chapter 2:
Frown Lines, Smile Lines,
and Other Lines of Expression

WHAT ARE THE DIFFERENT LINES OF EXPRESSION?
Frown Lines • Forehead Lines • Nasal Scrunch Lines • Crow's-Feet •
Creases at the Base of the Nose • Lip Lines • Chin Dimpling

WHAT ARE THE POSSIBLE TREATMENTS?
Botox • Collagen • Other Filler Agents • Facial Liposculpture •
Laser Resurfacing • TCA Peels

Part II: COLOR PROBLEMS

Part IV: SKIN HEALTH AND SUNSCREEN

Part V: COMMON SKIN PROBLEMS

APPENDIX

Acknowledgments

My husband, Mark, and I owe many, many thanks to all the people who helped bring this book into existence: to Hay House for seeing its possibilities; to Jean Naggar for representing us; to Larry Taubman for his guidance; to Suzanne Duroux for her help shaping this project; to the best co-workers in the world—Amy Sarkie, Mary Lorentsen, Jane Otway, Patty Perkins, Lisa Kelley, and Rochelle Manuel—who not only gave input on the book but have made Madison Skin and Laser what it is; to Dr. John Olerud, Chairman of Dermatology at the University of Washington, for his understanding; to our friends and colleagues at Hillis Clark Martin and Peterson for their tolerance; to Brant, Gavin, and Zan for their interest and patience; to Frances McPherson for the encouragement and generosity that gave us the breathing room to undertake this; and most important of all, to Brenda Partridge for her incredible skills, commitment, and work ethic—which she gave to us on her own time.

ෙ ෙ ෙ   ෙ ෙ ෙ

INTRODUCTION

Your Best Face provides solid medical information that can help you look vital and attractive for your age. I hope that it will enhance your own unique beauty, style, and sexuality, no matter how old you are. Getting older may bring a few lines to your face, but it can also make you more comfortable with yourself as you appreciate that you have a whole new type of wisdom and beauty.

OUR OWN BEAUTY: MY PHILOSOPHY

I believe that all people are beautiful, whether we have black, blonde, red, or chestnut hair; generous or slim figures; ebony, olive, or ivory skin. The important thing is to understand and be confident in our own beauty, in our own unique way, with our own sense of style.

Beauty is so much more than a two-dimensional image on the front of a magazine—it's a wonderful and unpredictable blend of confidence, inner strength, physicality, sensuality, facial features, spirit, and personality. After all, each one of us has

met physically beautiful people who seemed to become uninteresting and plain over time because their inner qualities didn't match their exteriors; conversely, we know people who initially didn't seem attractive to us but who grew beautiful because of who they were.

Think, for example, of CNN correspondent Christiane Amanpour, Andrea Jung (the CEO of Avon), Oprah Winfrey, Jennifer Lopez, or Rosie O'Donnell—none of these women look alike, and yet they're all beautiful. They're beautiful because of their vitality, their confidence, and their comfort with who they are, which enhances their physical beauty.

My hope is that this book will help your exterior match the confidence and energy that you're already developing within yourself.

A DERMATOLOGIST'S POINT OF VIEW

In a perfect world, we could all act with confidence and comfort in our own skin regardless of our appearance, but realistically, we create impressions partly because of how we look. Many women tell me that they feel more youthful than the person they see in the mirror. They feel younger than their chronological age, and they want to match that image in the mirror with their inner reality, which is more youthful and vital. They don't want to look decades younger, and they dislike that stretched look that occurs after some types of plastic surgery. Advances in modern dermatology have helped make gentler improvements in skin a reality.

Everywhere I go, I meet women who are eager for reliable information about skin. For instance, a friend once invited me to dinner with a number of her acquaintances. When one of the women discovered that I was a dermatologist, she asked me a question about collagen. As I opened my mouth to reply, I noticed that every woman at the table was straining to hear what I had to say—and soon they were all chiming in with their own questions.

At my clinic in Seattle, I practice both cosmetic and medical dermatology, and I see many patients who want to know what modern dermatology can do to improve their skin. And the questions I'm asked aren't just about collagen or Botox. Women wonder if Retin-A and topical vitamin C really work; they want trustworthy advice on sunscreens for themselves and their children; they want to know if lasers can really reverse sun damage with very little downtime. They ask questions about peels, microdermabrasion, and laser photorejuvenation: *Exactly what are these treatments for? What's involved in the treatment? How much downtime do they require? How much do they cost?*

And so, I was inspired to write *Your Best Face* (along with my husband, Mark), in order to (1) share useful, trustworthy information on how to have healthier, more beautiful skin; (2) cover, in a straightforward and practical way, the latest treatments developed by modern medical dermatology; and (3) answer the many questions I hear every day from my patients, who all want the best possible skin.

૭૭   ૭૭   ૭૭

ANSWERING YOUR QUESTIONS

This book gives me the opportunity to answer the questions women have asked me for years, and I've structured the chapters to address these questions. Each chapter gives you the basic causes of a particular skin problem, the treatments for it, and a discussion of the problem in a question-and-answer format.

- **Part I covers wrinkles,** from the early, fine wrinkles of our late 20s and 30s; to the frown lines, smile lines, and forehead lines of facial expressions; to the deeper creases of our 40s, 50s, 60s, and 70s. These chapters also include detailed discussions of laser photorejuvenation, microdermabrasion, Botox, and collagen. The last chapter in Part I covers lasers in general, and explains how to find a good cosmetic dermatologist and laser center.

- **Part II deals with color problems.** Here you can read about brown spots and age spots, blotchiness, and skin that's too red. Treatments for these color problems include lasers, bleaching creams, prescription medication, and also lifestyle changes.

- **Part III discusses texture problems,** including lumps, bumps, and moles; unwanted hair; scars; and oily or dry complexions that have different issues with pore size and texture. I also discuss cleansers and moisturizers here, along with some of the topical vitamin creams now available.

- **Part IV focuses on skin health and problem prevention.** Here I discuss nutrition, diet, certain health issues, and sunscreens.

- **Part V concentrates on acne, rosacea, and sensitive and allergic skin,** three very common skin diseases that I'm often asked about.

Since some of you may go directly to the topics that interest you the most, you may find some repetition. For example, some of the information on lasers in Chapters 1, 3, and 4 also appears in later chapters on brown spots and blotchiness. I want you to be able to dip in and read about the things you care most about—don't worry about reading the entire book from cover to cover.

෨෨ ෨෨ ෨෨

Please understand that this isn't a book denigrating plastic surgery. I work with many excellent plastic surgeons whom I respect immensely. There are definitely certain problems for which plastic surgery is still the best option—for example, excess skin on the upper eyelid, or skin that hangs down significantly below the jawline. But there are many skin problems for which there are other options besides surgery—those that allow us to improve our skin while continuing our busy lives. This book is about *all* of those options.

I want to give you something far more substantial than the promise of some magic cream or lotion; instead, I'd like to give you the most complete, up-to-date information on how to look your best. Keep in mind that knowing about and caring for your skin is the first step to keeping it healthy—because healthy skin is beautiful skin, which can help give you confidence. Whether you're a hard-working parent, nurse, doctor, CEO, entrepreneur, or teacher, appreciating the health and beauty of your skin will translate into feeling better about yourself, which in turn will enhance every area of your life.

Styles change, but humans will always greet the world face first. Why not present *your best face?*

— Brandith Irwin & Mark McPherson
www.yourbestface.net

ରତ ରତ ରତ   ରତ ରତ ରତ

PART I

WRINKLES

1

FINE WRINKLES

In the first three chapters of this book, I'm going to discuss wrinkles. Why three separate chapters? Wrinkles are just wrinkles, right? Well, for doctors who study and treat them, there *are* different kinds of wrinkles, which may call for different kinds of treatments.

I'm going to start by covering fine wrinkles—the tiny little lines that appear in our 20s to 40s, generally due to sun exposure. In this chapter, you'll find detailed information on popular treatments for fine wrinkles, such as microdermabrasion, peels, and photorejuvenation (a new, gentle laser treatment that treats fine lines and sun damage).

In the next chapter, I'll discuss crow's-feet; frown, lip, and forehead lines; and other types of wrinkles that are formed based on how we move the muscles of our face when we express ourselves. These so-called lines of expression usually appear in our 30s to 50s, and Botox is an increasingly popular treatment for them. Turn to this chapter for

answers to your many questions on Botox, as well as other treatments for lines of expression.

Chapter 3 covers deep wrinkles, the deeper creases that occur in our 40s to 70s, depending on our sun exposure, health habits, and age. Collagen can fill out and lift these deeper wrinkles, and you'll find a detailed section on collagen here. Laser resurfacing is also an option for deep wrinkles, and you can learn about that in this chapter as well.

And then in Chapter 4, I'll provide an overview of laser procedures and tell you how to find a good dermatologist and laser center.

In each chapter of this section (and in the rest of the book, too), I've included the most common questions I've received from my patients regarding each topic. I hope that you'll find answers to *your* questions as well.

Now, let's look at fine wrinkles, those first tiny lines that often appear around the mouth or on the cheeks. What causes them? And how can you smooth them out?

WHAT ARE THE POSSIBLE CAUSES?

(Please remember that there may be one or more causes for fine wrinkles, including some that may not be listed here.)

- Sun damage
- Dry conditions
- Weather
- Irritation from products

WHAT ARE THE POSSIBLE TREATMENTS?

We're all individuals, so there may be variations in treatment depending on your particular needs and your doctor's style of practice. Here are some of the most common:

- Moisturizers
- Laser photorejuvenation
- Microdermabrasion
- Light and "chemical" peels

POSSIBLE CAUSES

Fine Wrinkles on the Face

"What are fine wrinkles, and what causes them?"

Fine lines or wrinkles are those tiny, almost imperceptible lines that tend to start appearing in our 20s. Rather than forming deep creases, they tend to spread out and give the skin an uneven texture, almost like crepe paper. Fine wrinkles often appear around the eyes or on the cheeks starting in our 30s or 40s. These fine lines tend to appear due to one or more of the following:

Sun damage. Most of us grow up thinking that wrinkles are a natural part of aging. In fact, most of the wrinkles on our faces are actually due to sun damage and poor health habits—not aging. If you have trouble believing this, just stand in front of a mirror and look at your face, neck, and chest—or the back of your hands—which haven't been protected from the sun, and then look at your breasts, which have. My guess is that you'll see many more tiny wrinkles on the sun-exposed areas if you're over 30. And if you're not, you still have sun damage—you just aren't seeing the results of it yet. Also, while eating healthfully is important, consuming sugar isn't what causes wrinkles. If that were the case, your *entire body* would be wrinkled, not just the sun-exposed areas.

Sunlight is more complicated than you might think. The first step to avoiding more sun damage is to think "light" instead of "sunlight," because all natural light contains ultraviolet radiation. It's just that different times of the day and year, geographic locations, and weather all affect the amount of light radiation that you're getting. You'll get higher doses of skin-damaging ultraviolet radiation during the middle of the day, on sunny days, during the months closer to the June summer solstice, at higher altitudes, and on the water and snow.

You need to think about where you are and what you're doing to save your skin from further sun damage. While UVB light radiation peaks during midday, UVA radiation, which is just as damaging in the long run but doesn't usually cause a sunburn, is present all day long. UVA also damages your skin through window glass, the windshield of your car, and clouds. So think protection from *light,* not *sunlight!* You'll need ample protection from both UVB *and* UVA radiation.

To protect yourself against sun damage, wear sunscreen daily and "think zinc." Apply a zinc-containing sunscreen of at least SPF 20 on your face, neck, and chest every single morning. It doesn't hurt to put it on your hands and arms, also.

Here's how to do it: Clean your skin, and then apply the zinc-containing sunscreen. Use one in a moisturizing base if you're dry; if you're oily, use one in a drier base (you may need guidance from your dermatologist if you're having trouble). The sunscreen may be moisturizing enough that you don't need a separate moisturizer; if you need a little extra, apply it afterwards. Be sure to put on enough sunscreen—at least a teaspoon to cover your face and neck—since applying too little won't protect you.

How to Choose a Sunscreen

You'll need three sunscreens: one for daily use for your face, neck, chest, and hands; one for outdoor sports, vacations, and other high-sun activities; and one for your body.

1. First, pick a daily sunscreen for your face, which blocks both UVA and UVB rays. You'll put this on every morning after you wash your face, under anything else (such as foundation or moisturizer). Try Cetaphil Daily Facial Moisturizer SPF 15 (sold in drugstores), SkinCeuticals Daily Sun Defense SPF 20 or 30 (found in dermatologists' offices), Clinique City Block SPF 15 or Super City Block SPF 25 (sold in department stores), Olay Complete UV Defense Moisture Lotion (sold in drugstores), or M.D. Forté Environmental Protection Cream SPF 30 (found in dermatologists' offices).

2. Second, for your face, neck, and chest especially, pick a sunscreen for high-sun situations, such as vacations, swimming, and other outdoor sports and activities. Invest in a really good one that has at least 4 to 7 percent zinc, is waterproof, sweatproof, and SPF 30 or above. Try SkinCeuticals Sport SPF 45. (**Note:** These sunscreens can be expensive.)

3. Third, pick one for your body for times when you're outside swimming, working, or exercising but don't want to put the really expensive sunscreen all over your body. Try waterproof Coppertone Sport SPF 45 in the big bottle.

Remember, protective clothing is better than sunscreen. (See **www.sunprecautions.com**.)

Dry conditions. You may have already noticed that your fine lines show up more when your skin is dry. Water in the skin is important to keep skin cells and the spaces between them plumped up. The trick is to stay hydrated so that those water molecules are trapped in your skin. It's doubtful that being too dehydrated in itself causes wrinkles, but when the outer layers of the skin get too dry, the fine lines already there become more obvious. If you keep your skin well hydrated, you'll notice these lines less.

Even in a moist climate, such as the one I live in (Seattle), I see a dramatic increase in complaints of dry skin and eczema in October, when central heating starts being used. Central heating and air-conditioning systems blow dry, nonhumidified air into homes and work spaces. Many of us spend our time in these heated or air-conditioned climates, and the dryness of such environments makes wrinkles more visible. An especially low-humidity environment, such as an airplane, can really dry out the skin, and definitely aggravates the appearance of fine lines.

If you're not sure what fine wrinkles look like, try this experiment. Take some Ivory soap (a harsh cleanser that strips most of the oil off the skin) and wash your face twice with it. Don't apply any moisturizers

at all, and wait for anywhere from 30 minutes to two hours. You should be able to clearly see the appearance or aggravation of fine lines on your face.

Next, try washing your skin with a nondrying cleanser, such as Cetaphil, and then moisturize immediately afterwards. Look at the difference. You can try this experiment using Ivory and no moisturizer on one side of your face and Cetaphil with a moisturizer on the other side if you're still not convinced. This experiment shows you the difference between skin that's dry and stripped of its natural oils and skin that retains its water content in the outer layers. Remember that oil on your skin helps hold water in.

Allowing water to penetrate into the outer layers of the skin plumps it up. A good-quality moisturizer retains water by not letting it evaporate off the skin. Many modern moisturizers also contain ingredients called *humectants* that help bind water molecules and hold them in the skin longer.

The best way to hydrate the skin is to apply warm water to your face for several minutes, which will allow water to penetrate into the outer layers of your skin. While the skin is still damp, apply your moisturizer. If you have very dry skin or work in a low-moisture environment, then you may want to hydrate and moisturize more often than twice a day. Remember that good skin-care habits may not make a difference over a day or week—but over many years, the effects can be dramatic.

Weather. In addition to the sun, extremes of heat, cold, and wind also dry out the outer barrier layer of skin. Too much water evaporates out of the skin, making it look dry and accentuating fine lines.

Irritation from products. If your skin-care products are over-exfoliating or irritating you, your fine lines may appear worse. This situation is more common than you think, with so many products having alpha-hydroxy acids, vitamin-A derivatives, vitamin C, and many other potential irritants in them. Scrubs can be very rough on the skin—most of us shouldn't be using them more than once a week at most, especially if you're using other products that are potentially irritating. If you're not sure if irritation is part of your problem, take your products to your dermatologist and ask her to evaluate the situation. (**Please note:** I'll use the feminine pronoun for each usage from now on, even though your dermatologist may be male.)

Facial eczema. This is sometimes a lifelong problem, but it can also be caused by irritation or allergic reactions to products including soaps, lotions, moisturizers, cosmetics, shampoos, conditioners, and other hair products. The eye area is particularly prone to allergic problems. *Do not* try to treat this alone; you'll need help from your dermatologist.

Fine Wrinkles on the Neck and Chest

"I'm in my late 30s, and my face looks pretty good—but I've noticed that I'm developing fine lines on my neck and upper chest. What can I do to prevent these from deepening into wrinkles?"

Just as with the face, a lot of the fine lines on the neck and chest are primarily due to sun damage. Believe it or not, age is really a secondary factor for many types of wrinkles. I have patients in their 50s and 60s who have religiously used sun protection and who have almost no lines on their neck and chest; conversely, I have patients in their 20s and 30s who have had a lot of sun exposure and who already have fine wrinkles. Those fine lines will progress over time into deep wrinkles and that blotchy, leathery skin most of us would rather avoid.

Many of us are careful about sunscreen on our face but forget that our necks and upper chests are exposed much of the time, too. This is particularly true if you live in a warmer climate, such as Southern California, Florida, or the Southwest. Even in areas such as Seattle or New York, UVA radiation penetrates clouds and windows . . . and those of us who live in cloudy or wintry climates often overdo the sun when it does come out.

I strongly recommend getting in the habit of putting a good-quality sunscreen on your face, neck, chest, and backs of the hands every morning. That might sound ridiculous, but even in a rainy climate, many of us are exposed to more light than we think. Sure, we're only exposed to a small amount of radiation daily, but over 365 days a year, year after year, the math is impressive.

If you apply sunscreen as part of your morning routine, it will become a habit. And you won't get caught unprepared when the day suddenly turns sunny or you end up being outside more than you thought you'd be. If you live in a dark, cloudy city, just be sure that you're getting enough vitamin D (from dairy products, calcium supplements, or multivitamins) so that you don't become deficient. Vitamin D is made in the skin upon exposure to light, and it's important to keep your bones strong.

Fine Lines Around the Eye Area

"I just turned 30, and I'm noticing lines appearing around my eyes. Is there anything I can do about this?"

Many of us notice fine wrinkles around or under our eyes before any other place on our face. The skin around the eye area tends to be thinner than on other parts of the face, it contains fewer oil (sebaceous) glands, and we move this area a great deal when we use various facial expressions. In addition, as we get older, there's loss of elasticity from sun damage, and, in some of us, loss or slippage of the fat pad under the skin in that area.

What can you do? First of all, prevent any more sun damage by using a nonirritating sunscreen around your eye area in the morning. A good one to try is Dermalogica Total Eye Care SPF 15. You can also use your regular moisturizer and then put a nonirritating sunscreen around the eye area. Don't put the sunscreen right up to the eyelid margin, because it may sting if it gets in the eye. If your skin will tolerate it, you could try one with a low percentage of alpha-hydroxy acid in it to boost cell-turnover rate (M.D. Forté makes several of these). Again, this won't make a difference in a week or a month, but over several months, you should see some improvement.

A carbon dioxide or erbium laser peel (explained later in the chapter) will also give you excellent results around the eyes. But this is only an option if your skin isn't very sun damaged—otherwise, the skin around the eyes will look fresher and lighter in color, creating a mismatch with the rest of your face that's still sun damaged. You'll end up looking a little like a raccoon. Some excellent dermatologists will use the laser around the eyes and then a TCA peel on the rest of the face to make sure you're even.

POSSIBLE TREATMENTS

Moisturizers

"Is there any cream I can buy that will get rid of the wrinkles that I'm beginning to develop?"

I know you wish that all those claims in the advertisements were true, but no skin cream can get rid of all or even most of your wrinkles. However, a fairly substantial body of science now supports the use of some creams to treat fine wrinkles caused by sun damage.

The gold standard is still Renova or Retin-A. These are both *tretinoin* (the term for the generic compound). More scientific data supports the use of tretinoin to improve sun-damaged skin than any other product on the market, but unfortunately, this vitamin-A derivative still requires a prescription. Renova is tretinoin in a richer, more emollient base made for older skins, while Retin-A is a "drier" cream formulated more for oilier skins and acne. Tretinoin now also comes in generic forms that are cheaper. The only downside is that you may not know what type of base it's in.

A great deal of confusion exists about Renova/Retin-A/tretinoin versus retinol, which is available now in many over-the-counter skin creams. Retinol is converted to tretinoin by enzymes in the skin in very small amounts. Using retinol in a cream is like using a very weak version of Renova. Its only advantage is that it's less irritating for people who find that Renova causes too much peeling and redness.

There's also quite a large body of data supporting the use of alpha- and beta-hydroxy acids (such as glycolic or salicylic acid). Topical vitamin C in the form of L-ascorbic acid also has reasonable data to support its use. (See Chapters 9 and 12 for more information.)

Unfortunately, there are many other products on the market now that have very limited or no data to support their inflated sales pitches. Remember, anyone can market something as a *cosmeceutical* (as opposed to a drug) and claim pretty much whatever they want. All the company has to prove is that it won't hurt you—it doesn't have to prove that it really works. There are many "anti-aging" creams in this category, such as Kinerase, alpha-lipoic acids, "vitamin C ester" (as opposed to L-ascorbic acid), and retinol. There are no good-quality, double-blinded, placebo studies of these products with 100 or more patients, so these are interesting products that may in the future be supported by good data . . . but right now, they're supported mostly by marketing hype.

Moisturizers in and of themselves are very helpful if you have fine lines. A good moisturizer can be as simple as Cetaphil cream, Vanicream, or Olay Beauty Fluid, which can be found in most drugstores. There are also excellent products in your dermatologist's office. Some salons carry moisturizers that contain a number of new (but as yet unproven) vitamins, botanical extracts, and extracts from marine algae and so forth. Basic moisturizers work well even if they're not always cosmetically elegant. The expense of a moisturizer is sometimes more related to its spreadability, fragrance, and other cosmetic factors than its ability to help your skin retain moisture.

ඐ   ඐ   ඐ

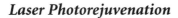

How to Choose a Good Moisturizer

You'll need two moisturizers: one for morning (with sunscreen in it), and one for bedtime (without sunscreen). Many moisturizers now also contain renewal products, such as vitamins and antioxidants, but save these mostly for nighttime. Never sacrifice using your sunscreen for a renewal product.

1.   First, pick a moisturizer for your face with sunscreen that blocks both UVA and UVB rays. You'll put this on every morning after you wash your face, under anything such as foundation or moisturizer. Try Cetaphil Daily Facial Moisturizer SPF 15 (sold in drugstores), SkinCeuticals Daily Sun Defense SPF 20 or 30 (found in dermatologists' offices), Clinique City Block SPF 15 or Super City Block SPF 25(sold in department stores), Olay Complete UV Defense Moisture Lotion (sold in drugstores), or MD Forte Environmental Protection Cream SPF 30 (found in dermatologists' offices).

2.   Second, choose your night moisturizer. Use your renewal product (such as Renova, topical vitamin C, alpha-hydroxy acids, and so on) first on clean skin and let it dry for a few minutes. Then, if you still feel dry, put on a little moisturizer. Try SkinCeuticals Hydrating B5 Gel (found in dermatologists' offices), Cetaphil Moisturizing Lotion or Cream (sold in drugstores), or Neutrogena Visibly Firm Night Cream (sold in drugstores).

Laser Photorejuvenation

"I'm in my 30s, but I've had a lot of sun damage. Now I'm getting wrinkles. Is there anything I can do for this besides moisturize?"

Yes. There's a very gentle laser technique called *photorejuvenation,* which is remarkably helpful for sun-damaged skin and may help reduce fine wrinkles as well. This treatment can be done in your dermatologist's office in about 30 to 60 minutes. The very gentle laser light doesn't break the skin at all. After the treatment, you can reapply makeup (if you want) and go right back to work.

Over a series of treatments, laser photorejuvenation removes or reduces many of the visible signs of sun damage, such as redness, broken and dilated blood vessels, age spots and brown spots, and in many cases, fine lines.

"How does photorejuvenation improve the appearance of sun-damaged skin and increase collagen production?"

The laser emits a very specific beam of light at a wavelength that targets *hemoglobin* (the pigment of red blood cells) or *melanin* (the brown pigment found in freckles and age spots). The laser beam passes through the skin and is absorbed by either hemoglobin or melanin. This damages the vessel wall or fragments the melanin pigment. These damaged vessels and the melanin pigment are then absorbed by the body and rendered less visible.

Studies have also shown that the laser light stimulates certain cells (*fibroblasts)* in the deeper layers of the skin (the *dermis)* that make collagen, so they begin to make new collagen. Over a period of many months, this often results in smoother skin with fewer fine wrinkles.

"Are there any other benefits?"

Many patients notice a small reduction in their pore size, a decrease in rosacea symptoms such as flushing, and a general improvement in texture and color. In some parts of the country, particularly California, photorejuvenation is being used as a maintenance tool, with treatments given every one to six months. This is controversial because studies haven't been done to determine how long the increase in collagen production continues after a treatment. Many laser centers are currently recommending maintenance treatments every six months until better data becomes available.

Laser photorejuvenation does not help lines of expression (such as frown lines, smile lines, or early crow's-feet) or deeper lines around the mouth and chin. It may improve small, early lines around the lips, but it definitely doesn't afford much improvement to deep lines in that particular area.

"Do the treatments hurt?"

There may be mild discomfort during the treatments, but you'll be able to tolerate them very easily. For discomfort, you may want to use a numbing cream (such as lidocaine), which you would apply approxi-

mately one hour before and again 20 minutes before a treatment. Your dermatologist will advise you.

If you're someone whose skin is bright red and has many dilated blood vessels, there will be a lot for the laser to target, so the first several treatments may be moderately uncomfortable. Try taking acetaminophen the night before and the morning of your treatments. Your dermatologist may also have suggestions to make you comfortable.

"How long do the treatments take?"

It varies, depending on the size of the treatment area. If you're just having your face treated, 30 to 60 minutes is common. Adding the neck and chest takes more time.

"How are the treatments done?"

When you come to the laser center, you'll be shown to a "laser room." Special glasses or eye pads will protect your eyes. A cold gel will then be placed on the skin being treated. The smooth glass surface of the handpiece will be gently applied to your skin, and pulses of light will be applied. You may feel a slight sting, like the snapping of a small rubber band. At the end of the treatment, the gel will be wiped off, the area will be cleaned with a warm cloth, and moisturizer will be applied. If there's any swelling, you might be given a cold pack to apply for ten minutes or so. Most centers will let you reapply foundation or concealer immediately after a treatment.

"How many treatments will I need?"

The average number of treatments to effectively remove broken blood vessels or age spots/freckles and increase collagen production is five. (However, some patients may require more or less than that.) Treatments are usually performed three to four weeks apart, but the interval may be longer. Multiple treatments are usually given over several months, with gradual clearing occurring over that time. Expect to start noticing improvements after the third treatment—the effects may be seen before that but not always. Reduction of your fine wrinkles and increased smoothness of the skin usually becomes evident even later and may not be noticeable for six months to a year because the changes in collagen deeper in the skin are slower to occur.

"Is there anything I should avoid doing before my treatment?"

Try not to take aspirin, ibuprofen, or naproxen the week prior to your treatments because they'll make you slightly more likely to bruise. If you're taking these medications for medical reasons, ask your primary-care doctor first to make sure it's okay to stop. Anticoagulants such as Coumadin should be discussed with your dermatologist, who may want you to stop using other things as well, such as extra vitamin E, alcohol, St. John's wort, and Ginkgo biloba.

"Are there any restrictions on my activity right after the treatment?"

The only common restriction is exercise. You may be asked to refrain from vigorous exercise or yoga for several days after the treatment. Stay out of the sun; if you must go out in it, use a good sunscreen and a hat. (Your doctor will have specific instructions for you.)

"What will I look like right after the treatment?"

If you're being treated mostly for texture problems and fine wrinkles, you may not see any changes immediately after the treatment, for the changes take place deep in the skin where the collagen is made.

If you have dilated blood vessels or are red, expect a slightly sunburned look after the treatment for two to five days. There may even be mild to moderate puffiness for a day or two. Occasionally there's bruising, which can take up to two weeks to resolve.

If you're being treated for brown spots or freckling, they'll look darker for about a week—sometimes looking like tiny specks of dirt for several days—and then they'll gradually flake off. Makeup can usually be used right after the treatment as long as it's applied and removed very gently. Discuss this with your doctor first.

"What does laser photorejuvenation cost?"

This depends a lot on the area of the country where you live. The average cost for one treatment of the entire face is approximately $500—adding the neck, chest, or other areas will be more expensive. Some centers charge more for that extra pass over the skin with a longer wavelength to stimulate collagen production, which is sometimes referred to as the "wrinkle setting."

"Is there anyone who shouldn't have these treatments?"

Your doctor may advise against it if you're taking anticoagulants, medications, or antibiotics that heighten photosensitivity, or if you have a history of bleeding disorders. Be sure to discuss any health issues and medications with your dermatologist at the consultation.

"Are there any complications with this kind of treatment?"

Complications are rare, but they do occasionally occur. They can include the following:

- *Discomfort.* There may be a burning sensation that lasts for an hour or two.

- *Blistering.* There's always a slight possibility of developing a crust or blister. This is superficial and generally doesn't result in any scarring; it's treated like a sunburn or any other blister.

- *Pigment changes.* The treated area will probably heal without any pigment changes; however, there's always a chance that darker or lighter areas may crop up. These are usually temporary and will fade within one to six months. Sun exposure must be avoided if a darker spot occurs, as that may intensify the hyperpigmentation. It's rare that a change is permanent.

- *Scarring.* This is very rare if all post-treatment instructions are followed carefully.

- *Swelling.* This may occur immediately after treatment, especially on the face. It's temporary and not harmful.

Microdermabrasion

"Some of my friends have had microdermabrasion, and they look great. But is it safe?"

Microdermabrasion is actually a safe and gentle "light" peel and works well for mild to moderate sun damage, early fine lines, some melasma, mild acne that isn't inflamed, and oily skin. In my opinion, it isn't effective for acne scarring, but there's debate about this. It's also an excellent skin-maintenance tool after a gentle laser photorejuvenation series, trichloroacetic acid peels (TCA), or laser resurfacing.

Microdermabrasion has, to some extent, replaced glycolic and salicylic acid peels in many dermatologists' offices. There may be some situations where your doctor feels a glycolic or salicylic acid peel is more appropriate. Also, for some patients with very oily, tough, acne-prone skin, microdermabrasion *and* a glycolic or salicylic acid peel might be used in combination. This should be done with a doctor's supervision.

"Just what is microdermabrasion?"

A jet of very fine crystals is vacuumed across the skin to remove dead and damaged skin cells, refine the texture and color of your skin, and help improve mild acne. It stimulates blood flow to the surface of the skin, which increases oxygenation and stimulates cell turnover and renewal. It *does not* help with deeper wrinkles or lines of expression. Light glycolic acid peels may be applied with microdermabrasion to increase the effects. You may have seen the terms *Parisian peel, Diamond peel,* or *lunchtime peel.* These all refer to the same process—microdermabrasion.

"How does it work?"

The machine usually resembles

a large vacuum cleaner and has a soft, contoured metal handpiece that looks like a large pen. This handpiece vacuums very fine crystals across the skin, which are then sucked immediately back up off the skin and into a separate container of used crystals. When the used-crystal container is full, the old ones are thrown away and replaced with new crystals. Crystals are never reused on another person, and the metal tip of the handpiece should be sterilized or thrown away after each use.

The better machines have a pressure gauge that allows the operator to dial the pressure up or down according to the goals of the treatment and the sensitivity of the person being treated. The skin is often stretched a little bit in the area being treated. Treatments usually last between 30 and 60 minutes, depending on the number of areas being treated and the goals of the treatment. There's usually a mildly uncomfortable stinging sensation during the session, but the treatment itself shouldn't be painful.

"How many treatments will I need?"

This is quite variable. If you already have good skin or are trying to maintain the results achieved with laser treatments or a TCA peel, for example, once a month or once a quarter might be enough. If you're using microdermabrasion as the primary treatment for mild sun damage, melasma, or mild acne, five to ten treatments might be recommended, with a maintenance schedule after that. It's also important to maintain

your skin in between treatments. Ask your dermatologist about the use of sunscreens, Retin-A, daily glycolic acid, or vitamin C. She can optimize your skin health home-care regimen for you.

"Do the treatments hurt? How long will they take?"

For microdermabrasion, there's a mild pulling sensation during the treatment, but most patients don't notice anything other than mild discomfort. The treatments usually take 30 to 60 minutes, depending on the size of the treatment area.

If treatments are uncomfortable for you, you may want to purchase some lidocaine cream (such as ELA-Max), which is applied 45 minutes and 20 minutes before a treatment. Your dermatologist can tell you where to get this cream.

"Is there a difference between microdermabrasion in salons, versus doctors' offices?"

The microdermabrasion machines sold to doctors' offices are generally more powerful than those sold to salons. Often the physician models will have a pressure pedal that can be used to dermabrade deeper in certain areas if needed. Many salons, however, do an excellent job if what is needed is only a light microdermabrasion—the key is to find an experienced aesthetician.

"What should I do before my treatment?"

Always check with your doctor. Many will want you to stop certain products for several days before a treatment.

"What should I expect after a treatment?"

Your skin should feel extremely smooth and be pink to slightly red for several days. The neck and chest are a bit more sensitive and will usually remain red longer than the face. There may also be some obvious peeling or flaking during the first week after microdermabrasion.

You'll also notice that your skin feels slightly drier. It's important to use very gentle cleansers and lots of moisturizer the first week or so after a treatment. Ask your dermatologist when she'd like you to resume your regular skin care. Dermatologists vary on when they'll want you to begin other products again. Be sure to wear a sunscreen every morning.

"What areas can be treated?"

Just about any area can be treated, but the face, neck, and chest are the most common. Other areas, such as the back (especially if you have acne), the arms, the backs of the hands (if sun damaged), and even areas on the legs or trunk can also be treated.

Some dermatology offices even have machines with a tiny tip that was developed just for the delicate eye area. Be sure that the aesthetician you're working with turns the pressure down so as not to traumatize the delicate tissue around the eye. If microdermabrasion is done correctly, it may also soften fine lines in this area over time.

"Why did my doctor recommend a series of treatments?"

As with other "light" peels, one treatment alone doesn't work very well for acne, mild sun damage, brown spots, or fine lines. Usually a series of five to ten treatments approximately one to three weeks apart, depending on how sensitive your skin is, will be recommended at first. After the initial series, a maintenance program anywhere from monthly to quarterly might be advised.

"Why should I use microdermabrasion for skin health maintenance?"

If you've already been protecting yourself from the sun using state-of-the-art products and your skin is in good shape, you might benefit from microdermabrasion as a maintenance tool to help preserve your gains. Depending on your skin type, monthly or quarterly treatments may be helpful in maintaining your skin. If you have very oily, tough, acne-prone skin, monthly treatments might be appropriate; whereas if your skin is very fine, thin, and sensitive, quarterly sessions might be plenty. Your dermatologist can help you figure out which would be best for you.

"Will it make me less red?"

No. In fact, it may make the redness worse. Microdermabrasion doesn't improve dilated blood vessels or redness, so if you have active rosacea or acne that's red or inflamed, it isn't advised. (Be sure to check with your dermatologist if you have these skin conditions to see what her recommendation would be.)

"Is there anyone who shouldn't use it?"

You shouldn't use microdermabrasion on skin that's inflamed, infected, or has open sores or cuts, or if you have active eczema or psoriasis on your face. If you have active rosacea or moderate to severe acne, it's best to avoid microdermabrasion until those conditions are brought under better control. Sometimes microdermabrasion will be recommended for certain types of acne. Comedonal acne, which is characterized by lots of whiteheads and blackheads, usually responds nicely; cystic or pustular acne, which is already red and inflamed, may get worse.

"How much does it cost?"

This varies quite widely by area, but the average cost per treatment is $100 to $200. If more areas than the face are treated, the cost will be higher. Treatments are often sold in packages of five to ten, with a discount associated with the package. This can be a cost-effective way to go because, in the beginning, microdermabrasion is often most successful in a series anyway.

Light and "Chemical" Peels

"What exactly is a light peel?"

Light peels are usually done with one of two acids: glycolic acid, which is derived from sugar cane, or salicylic acid.

Glycolic acid peels. These are light and generally safe peels, which can be used in strengths varying from 20 percent up to 70 percent. They're sometimes performed by a physician, but in most cases, they're low-risk and safe enough to be performed by a nurse or a well-trained aesthetician. Only personnel directly under a doctor's supervision should perform the higher strength peels (in the 50 and 70 percent range).

Like all "light" peels, one treatment has very little effect—the benefits really accrue over a series of treatments. Generally, anywhere from three to ten light peels in a series will be recommended, depending on the problem. For example, if glycolic peels are being recommended to improve moderately severe acne, a series of ten treatments might be appropriate. To treat very light sun damage in a 28-year-old, however, three to five peels might be recommended.

Here's the process for a peel. After arriving at the office, you'll probably be asked to wash your face very carefully and dry it before the peel is started. You should then be offered a comfortable place to lie down during the peel. The practitioner will paint on the glycolic solution with a fine brush, gauze, or Q-Tip fairly quickly so that all areas of the face develop at about the same time. The solution is then left on for several minutes. Glycolic peels are generally timed, and this can be important: Solution left on too long can cause unwanted side effects. Your dermatologist will decide with each treatment how many minutes are appropriate. There tends to be a very mild stinging sensation that usually goes away right after the peel is completed.

Glycolic peels generally need to be neutralized with a solution of sodium bicarbonate, which can be a little messy but isn't at all uncomfortable. Towels are often placed around the neck and face to absorb any excess liquid from the neutralizing solution. Then moisturizer and sunscreen are usually applied.

Expect to be a little red and have some slight scaliness or very fine peeling for several days or a week afterwards, depending on the strength of the peeling solution. You shouldn't have bright redness, pain, or blisters—if any of these things occur, be sure to call your doctor right away. Problems can arise even with these quite safe peels if the solution is too strong for your particular skin type. Most dermatologists will start with a low-strength solution and progress up through higher strengths as the treatments go on to make sure that they're safe.

If you have a darker skin type, be sure to go to someone very experienced, because this type of peel can cause temporary and (rarely) permanent darkening of the skin if it isn't done very carefully.

Dermatologists vary in their opinions on whether you should temporarily stop using other products, such as Renova or Retin-A, after a peel. My opinion is that if you're red and scaly, you should give your skin a rest (with the exception of sunscreen and moisturizers) until the peeling process is completed. Follow your particular dermatologist's recommendation since regimens can vary greatly.

Salicylic acid peels. Salicylic acid peels are similar to glycolic peels but they often come prepackaged in a standard strength. Many of them also have a built-in timer so that the solution itself stops developing at a certain point without a second neutralizing agent. This can be beneficial, since it prevents the solution from being accidentally left on too long. However, these aren't completely foolproof, and it's possible to get overpeeled or have too much absorption in one area versus another. Some peels also have a color indicator that changes color when the peel process is completed. Salicylic acid peels may be better for acne, as they seem to penetrate down into the follicles better where the acne plugs *(comedones)* form. As with glycolic peels, one salicylic peel will have very little effect, and they're usually performed in a series to achieve maximum effect.

Trichloroacetic acid "chemical" peels. These differ from glycolic and salicylic acid peels and microdermabrasion in that they're generally deeper. Trichloroacetic acid (TCA) can be used in concentrations anywhere from 15 to 40 percent (the most common are in the 20 to 35 percent range), which are considered medium-depth peels. A deep peel would be considered a carbon dioxide or erbium laser peel. A light to medium TCA peel might be used for fine wrinkling, especially around the eyes or on the neck. Deeper laser peels are really not appropriate just for fine wrinkling. They're usually reserved for deeper wrinkles or sometimes very mild acne scarring.

A gentle 15 or 20 percent TCA peel should give you a little to moderate improvement in the lines around the eye area. This peel requires approximately five to seven days' healing time.

Options for Sensitive Skin

"My skin always looks irritated and wrinkled, and I have eczema. What should I be using?"

You're probably allergic to some of the common ingredients in skin creams—usually preservatives, lanolin, or fragrances—but there could be a number of other possibilities as well. The medical term for this is *contact allergic dermatitis,* sometimes referred to as *eczema.*

There are many different degrees of sensitive skin: Some of us experience a small amount of irritation from a product once every couple of years; some unlucky others have reactions to almost every product that they try. Think about where you might fall in that continuum. If you're clearly on the severe end of the scale (that is, you're having reactions to many products), it's important to see your dermatologist for allergy testing.

Allergy testing is painless. Your doctor will place a small disc on your back with waterproof tape so that you can shower. The discs stay on for 48 to 72 hours and are then read back in your dermatologist's office by the doctor or a nurse once or twice.

Often your dermatologist will start with a standard test kit containing 24 of the most common *allergens* (things you might be allergic to). If these prove negative and you're still having problems, then your dermatologist may recommend further testing—perhaps even with a doctor who specializes in this type of allergic problem.

If, on the other hand, your reactions are mild and only occasional, you may want to do your own detective work to identify the products that don't agree with you. Here are some steps you might try:

1. Stop using all soaps and lotions.

2. Switch temporarily to Cetaphil skin cleanser and cream for a week or two. Keep in mind that you may be allergic to Cetaphil products, although this is unusual. (You can also try the "Free and Clear" line of Vani-cream products.) If Cetaphil is worsening your situation, then stop using it and call your dermatologist.

3. Try over-the-counter hydrocortisone in one-percent strength, but keep in mind that some people become allergic to this over time. If the hydrocortisone seems to be making the situation worse, then stop using it and call your dermatologist right away.

4. Once your skin has been back to normal for about a week, try adding your products back in one at a time, approximately four days to a week apart. See if you can identify which one causes the reaction.

5. If you know exactly which product it was, then don't ever use it again. It's helpful to save the labels of products that you've had bad experiences with. If your sensitivity seems to be getting worse over time, a good dermatologist can often read the labels of four or five products and narrow down the possible offenders fairly easily.

SUMMARY OF FINE WRINKLES: WHAT TO DO

Let's assume that your fine wrinkles are caused by the sun and weather, rather than allergies, extremely dry skin, or reactions to products. What should you do? Here's what I recommend:

- Use a good-quality **sunscreen** every morning on your face, neck, chest, and backs of the hands.

- Use scientifically proven **skin-renewal products** such as Renova, alpha- and beta-hydroxy acids, or topical vitamin C. Discuss these with your dermatologist first if you can.

- **Moisturize** your skin and keep it hydrated.

If you want to step up your efforts and spend more time and money to reduce your sun damage, here are the treatments that work best for most skin types:

- **Laser photorejuvenation**—be prepared for five treatments at approximately $500 per treatment for the face (the cost varies depending on your doctor and where you live).

- **Microdermabrasion**—a light peel that's done in a series of approximately five treatments at a cost of approximately $100 to $200 per treatment.

- **Light chemical peels**—a series of glycolic or salicylic acid peels may yield good results and, like microdermabrasion, are more affordable than laser photorejuvenation.

Be sure to discuss these treatments with your doctor so that you know the costs and risks for your particular skin type and situation.

๑๐ ๑๐ ๑๐   ๑๐ ๑๐ ๑๐

2

FROWN LINES, SMILE LINES, AND OTHER LINES OF EXPRESSION

Wrinkles don't just result from age or sun damage, they're also created by the way we express ourselves. Dermatologists call them "lines of expression"—wrinkles that form over time from scrunching noses, frowning, raising eyebrows, or merely talking and smiling.

Coco Chanel, the great fashion designer, once said that at age 18 we have the face that nature gives us, and after 40 we have the face that our life and character give us. In essence, she was saying that lines of expression give us individuality. Most of us want to keep that unique sense of character and life experience in our faces, yet we also want to apply modern dermatology in order to soften some of the lines that have become deeper and more pronounced than we like. Let's see how we can do that.

WHAT ARE THE DIFFERENT LINES OF EXPRESSION?

- Frown lines
- Forehead lines
- Nasal scrunch lines
- Crow's-feet
- Creases at the base of the nose
- Lip lines
- Chin dimpling

WHAT ARE THE POSSIBLE TREATMENTS?

- Botox
- Collagen
- Other filler agents
- Facial liposculpture
- Laser resurfacing or TCA peels

LINES OF EXPRESSION: ERASE OR RELAX?

Lines of expression are created by the way our faces move. Some of these include habits learned from our parents: Babies stare intently at their parents' faces and try to mimic their expressions; as children get older, they pick up certain gestures of their parents and siblings, which is partly why family members often resemble one another. Other expressions, such as smiling or frowning, seem to be hardwired into our individual makeup.

Whether expressions are based on mimicry or there's some genetic coding involved, they create wrinkles that form and deepen over time. And when you add sun damage and habits such as smoking, it's easy to see how these lines get more pronounced as we get older.

Our facial expressions are part of what makes us individuals. While everyone gets certain types of lines (such as crow's-feet around the eyes), the way they form is quite varied. When I work with these wrinkles, my goal is to help patients look like themselves, only more rested and relaxed—and perhaps a bit younger.

Personally, I think that trying to erase all lines of expression is a mistake. We've all seen people, particularly on Oscar night, who have so inhibited these lines of facial expression that their faces have an almost frozen, masklike appearance—this is *not* attractive to me. When I work with Botox, collagen, and other filler agents, my goal isn't to completely eliminate expression or to immobilize the face, but to soften the wrin-

kles. (The one exception is frown lines: Relaxing those muscles so that they don't move very much is usually quite beneficial, even to those of us who aren't actors.)

Frown Lines

"I'm only 30 years old, but I'm already starting to get frown lines. Should I start Botox now?"

It used to be that collagen was primarily used to lift frown lines out and make the area look smooth, but Botox has pretty much supplanted the use of collagen in this area. In fact, the most common use for Botox is to relax frown lines.

Of course, most people who have these kinds of lines aren't frowning deliberately. They've just developed a muscular habit over many years, and the tension that results is completely unconscious. Many of my Botox patients say that they get tired of people thinking, and sometimes asking, if they're angry or unhappy, when they actually feel fine. And so, the relaxation of these lines gives them a friendlier, more approachable look.

After using Botox consistently for six months to two years, it's unusual to still need collagen in that area. When Botox relaxes the muscle causing the frown line to form, the line usually fades away simply due to that action. Expect the process to take longer if your lines are deeper.

Since Botox has so many uses now, let's discuss it in detail with respect to frown lines first—then we'll tackle its use in other facial areas.

"What is Botox?"

Botox is a formulation of *botulinum toxin type A,* which is derived from a bacterium called *Clostridium botulinum.* Type A is just one of seven different forms of botulinum toxin, and each one has slightly different properties and actions. No two botulinum toxins are exactly alike.

"How does it work?"

Normally your brain sends electrical signals to your muscles to make them move. The electrical message runs from the nerve to the muscle via a chemical messenger at the end of the nerve called *acetylcholine.* Botox blocks the nerve ending from releasing acetylcholine, and as a result, the muscle movements stop or are greatly reduced. Your dermatologist will know how much Botox is needed to treat you effectively.

"Is it a new treatment?"

No. Botox has been used for more than ten years to treat thousands of patients worldwide. The health ministries of at least 70 countries have approved it, and it's been endorsed by the American Academy of Neurology and the National Institutes of Health since 1990. These groups originally approved Botox for use in many different medical conditions—its cosmetic uses came later. It was only recently that Allergan, the company that makes Botox, applied for and received specific cosmetic approval for it.

"How was Botox discovered?"

Botulinum toxins were first studied in the 1940s. In the 1960s, the muscle-relaxing properties of botulinum type A were studied for investigational use in realigning crossed eyes, and these early studies paved the way for treating cosmetic problems caused by overactive muscles.

Botox is now produced in controlled laboratory conditions and given in extremely small therapeutic doses. It has helped tens of thousands of people worldwide who have conditions caused by overactive muscles, such as *cervical distonia* (a condition that causes severe neck spasms and pain). It's also been used in many thousands of patients for the treatment of *blepharospasm,* a condition in which the eyelid muscles twitch uncontrollably. Botox relaxes the eyelid muscles and allows patients to open their eyes. These are just a few examples of the many medical uses of Botox.

"When should I start using Botox?"

This is an individual decision, and there are no reputable long-term scientific studies to help us neatly answer this question. Some dermatologists advocate very early use to prevent wrinkles from ever forming in the first place. Others, including myself, vote for waiting until wrinkles are beginning to form or are formed—otherwise, where do we draw the line? Should high school or college students be using it now to prevent wrinkles in their 40s? Most of us would disagree with that idea.

The other approach is to start using Botox at the first hint of a line, with the assumption that it will keep lines from forming in the first place.

The downside of this is that you're having to deal with treatments earlier in life—not to mention the time and money involved (Botox is moderately expensive).

Another issue is the remote possibility of developing a resistance to Botox. Although it's been used for more than ten years with few reports of resistance, recently some medical literature has suggested that resistance *can* develop in a very, very small minority of users. (Most of these patients were using much larger doses for medical reasons and weren't cosmetic patients.)

In my opinion, it makes sense to start using Botox when actual lines or wrinkles are visible, but not before that.

"Do injections hurt?"

When injected, Botox doesn't cause irritation or inflammation. Occasionally, patients complain that the fluid feels like a very mild sting, but the discomfort is gone within several minutes.

"How long does it take for Botox to work?"

The effects are usually noticed in the first 72 hours, but it may take up to ten days to work fully. The first set of injections may provide only a partial response (which isn't uncommon); complete relaxation may not occur until after the second set of injections.

"How long do the effects last?"

Most patients who receive Botox find that the effects of the injections last approximately three months in the first year. In the second and third years, effects may last a bit longer, even up to four to six months. To maintain maximal relaxation of the muscles injected, plan on receiving injections approximately every three to five months, but this all depends on how strong your muscles are and how deep the lines are. The treatment can be repeated as long as it's required. (Since everyone has individual needs, there's variability in the times mentioned above.)

"Where can I use Botox?"

Botox is primarily used to relax frown lines, forehead lines, and crow's-feet. Less commonly, though, it can be used to raise the eyebrows (by injecting small amounts just under them); make the eyes look a little wider (by injecting just under them); or in the chin area or at the corners of the mouth if certain muscle groups pull down there. It's sometimes used in the neck, and a few drops in the upper lip can sometimes soften lip lines. Ask your dermatologist if you're interested in working on these areas.

"Are there any side effects?"

Because only small doses are used for facial wrinkling, no serious side effects have been reported. Rarely, a slight drooping of an eyelid can occur—if this happens, it usually resolves itself over a two- to eight-week period. If Botox is injected into the neck, the neck muscles themselves, or those in the voice box (the larynx), could become weak, which can result in temporary difficulty in speaking. In very, very rare instances, a resistance to Botox can develop.

A very small amount of bruising with Botox injections is fairly common and normal. Most dermatologists and their staff are proficient at avoiding noticeable blood vessels, but since there are so many tiny ones all over the face, bleeding can occur at any injection site. Bruises are generally small and last from three to ten days. They can be covered with makeup.

"Who shouldn't receive Botox?"

It shouldn't be given to pregnant women, nursing mothers, or people who have myasthenia gravis or other muscle diseases.

"How much does it generally cost?"

The cost of treatments varies widely by geographical area. For instance, treatments are usually more expensive in large cities such as New York and Los Angeles. Costs also vary depending on the number of areas on the face or neck being treated. The average treatment in most large cities is between $300 and $1,000. However, treating multiple areas—such as frown lines, crow's-feet, and horizontal forehead lines all in the same treatment—will boost your cost up toward the higher end. If you're just having frown lines treated, the cost should be closer to the low end.

"Is there anything I shouldn't do before my Botox treatment?"

Your doctor may ask you to avoid aspirin, ibuprofen (Advil), naproxen (Aleve), extra vitamin E, alcohol the night before, and any herbal preparations that "thin" the blood (inhibit clotting), such as St. John's wort and Ginkgo biloba, as they make bruising more likely. But talk to your doctor first if you're taking any medications for strokes, heart problems, and so on. (Coumadin, for example, is usually a medication that can't be stopped.) It's perfectly safe to have Botox injected even if you need to stay on one of these medications— you'll just be slightly more likely to have bruises.

The week prior to Botox treatment, acetaminophen may be taken for minor aches and pains without any problem.

"What about after my treatment?"

Dermatologists have different opinions on this, so be sure ask your own doctor. In general, though, stay upright and don't exercise for 4 or 5 hours, and don't stand your head or do yoga for 24 hours. It helps to frown or scrunch the muscles that were just treated several times an hour for an hour or two, for Botox binds better to active muscle. Some dermatologists prohibit flying for 24 hours due to changes in cabin pressure.

"Should I go to a Botox party?"

Botox parties are a new trend in which several people gather at one location (often medical offices or "medispas") to receive assembly-line Botox injections by one doctor or nurse. Botox is a medical procedure, and I think that medical care at its best is individual, intimate, and high quality—none of which are offered at these "parties." Here's more on why I think they're a bad idea:

— The best Botox is carefully individualized for you by a doctor; at a party, you'll get "McBotox," where everyone gets the same few shots in the forehead.

— The best Botox is part of a complete and unified approach to your sun-damage issues and skin problems, which you won't get at a party.

— Botox treatment should be intimate: During treatment at a dermatologist's office, many patients will ask other questions about their skin, and the answers are personal. You won't get the benefit of this extra care at a Botox party.

— The best Botox is safe and done in a high-quality environment. Botox is a very safe medication, and adverse reactions are very rare and usually temporary, but they still do occur occasionally. Why take the risk of having it injected in a party setting, where both you and the doctor might not be completely focused on the medical side? And adding alcohol to these parties may increase risks.

— Botox parties are marketing gimmicks. A doctor having a Botox party is trying to generate more business. Why? The best doctors are usually busy and don't need to rely on parties to build their practices. They rely on referrals from their happy patients and other doctors.

Forehead Lines

"I have deep lines in my forehead from raising my eyebrows when I talk. Would Botox help?"

The muscle that you're working when you raise your eyebrows is called the *frontalis,* and lines do result from overuse of that muscle.

The wrinkles start out as fine, almost imperceptible lines, and then they gradually get deeper and deeper as the muscle habit becomes more entrenched over time.

Botox is wonderful for deep horizontal forehead lines. It's injected in six to twelve small injections going all the way across the forehead—the number of injections depends upon how wide your forehead is, how strong the muscles are, and how much movement you want restricted. Usually when Botox is used on the entire forehead, the frown lines at the center (called the *glabella* area) are treated, also. (Of course, your dermatologist will customize your Botox treatment for your individual needs.)

This is a very safe area to treat with Botox. The only rare complication is an occasional temporary droopy eyelid or eyebrow on one side or the other. Again, this is very unusual if an experienced dermatologist is treating you. Small, temporary bruises are common.

Also, if you're over 40 and have a bit of excess skin hanging down over your eye on your upper eyelid, sometimes the entire brow will move down a little bit as the forehead relaxes and will make the excess skin from the eyelid more prominent. If you have that problem, Botox can be injected a little farther up on the forehead so that the muscles continue to lift in the area right around the eyebrow. Or a little Botox can be injected just under the eyebrow to lift the brow up—then the excess skin won't seem to hang down over the eye any differently than it did before the Botox. The other option is to have a good plastic surgeon surgically remove that excess skin. This is called an *upper lid blepharoplasty.*

When plastic surgeons do what's known as a *brow lift,* they sometimes cut the nerves to certain muscles in the forehead so that they can't contract. If you're having a brow lift for other reasons, you may want to discuss this with your plastic surgeon, for this is a permanent solution that can leave the forehead looking very flat with no movement at all. The advantage of Botox, even though it has to be repeated, is that it can be customized to allow some movement of the forehead and a more natural appearance over time.

Nasal Scrunch Lines

"I have wrinkles running across the bridge of my nose and down the sides. What causes these?"

These are called "nasal scrunch lines" (also referred to as "bunny" or "wolf" lines) and describe the lines that come from wrinkling up the nose. We all scrunch our nose, usually when we smell something bad, but some of us scrunch it repeatedly and form deep lines across the bridge or sides. The main muscle involved is called the *procerus muscle.* Botox works very well in this area and can be injected right into the muscle to relax those lines.

Crow's-Feet

"I seem to be getting more lines around my eyes. Would Botox help with this problem?"

Definitely—in fact, one of the best uses for Botox is on crow's-feet. A small amount is usually injected multiple times from about the end of the eyebrow down to about a half an inch below the eye. The site of the lowest injection depends on where your crow's-feet are, since each person is an individual. Injections here smooth this area nicely. Botox can be individualized for you, so if you'd like to retain some movement in the area so that it looks more natural, just let your dermatologist know.

The only downside to injecting this area, other than small bruises, seems to be a slight increase in the tiny wrinkles under the eye. Since the muscles lateral to the eye aren't working quite as hard and scrunching the way they normally do in a smile, in a few people there's a slight increase in puffiness below the eye. Sometimes that can be corrected by injecting a little higher up. This doesn't happen to everyone; also keep in mind that undereye puffiness is affected as much by salt intake, dehydration, PMS, allergies, and lack of sleep as by Botox injections.

Collagen can also be injected into crow's-feet (particularly if the wrinkles are deep), but it can be lumpy. Botox is usually recommended now, because collagen is often no longer needed after Botox relaxes the muscle under the wrinkle. If, after using Botox, there are still fairly pronounced lines, collagen may be used to fill those in a little bit. The skin is thin in this area, so collagen must be used carefully and sparingly to avoid leaving tiny lumps.

---⟡---

Get the Most Out of Your Botox

1. Frown or contract the muscles injected two or three times an hour for
    several hours after your Botox because it binds better to active muscle.

2. Schedule your next treatment when you see that the Botox is starting to
    wear off. If you wait until it's completely worn off, the muscles have a
    chance to get stronger again, and you won't receive the cumulative effect.

3. Most people find that keeping to a schedule allows the interval between
    treatments to gradually get longer. For example, a common schedule
    might be every three months the first year and then every four months
    the second year—some lucky people can eventually even go five or six
    months between treatements.

---⟡---

Creases at the Base of the Nose

"I'm developing a deep groove or fold that starts at the base of my nose. Is there anything I can do?"

Doctors call this the *nasolabial fold*. It starts at the base of the nose and creates a groove running down to the chin area. In some people, this fold is very pronounced; in others, it's quite minimal. A prominent fold here is usually an inherited tendency—look at your other family members. Options for treatment of this area are collagen, other filler agents such as fat and gortex, and facial liposculpture.

Collagen. Collagen and other filler agents are really the best treatment for this area. Botox usually isn't advisable here, because to relax the muscles around the nose and cheeks causes strange expressions when talking and eating. It would look a little bit as if you've had a mild stroke. Since no one wants a droopy mouth, collagen and other filler agents are the best treatment. The one exception would be the "marionette" lines that pull directly down at the corners of the mouth—a small amount of Botox here can sometimes lift up the corners of the mouth if that muscle is too strong.

Collagen works quite well around the mouth and nose. It's easy to use and can fill in all types of wrinkles, lines, and folds, and it does an excellent job of lifting the corners of the mouth. It's usually injected along the nasolabial fold and in wrinkles that extend around the mouth ("smile lines"). It can also be injected into the lines at the corners of the mouth, as well as other lines and creases on the cheeks.

Temporary bruising sometimes occurs, but the only way you can be harmed by collagen is if you're allergic to it. Most dermatologists will now allergy test *twice* before allowing you to start treatment. Each test is followed by a wait of approximately three to six weeks to observe for reactions. After the two tests, you have approximately a 90-percent chance of having no problems with collagen. Even if you've had collagen at another office, if it's been more than six months or a year, most doctors will still want to test you again.

There's the occasional unlucky person who, despite two allergy tests, will have a delayed reaction to the collagen. This reaction (which usually results in red, tender, itchy lumps at the injection sites) can be very unpleasant but will almost always resolve over a three- to six-month period. Anti-inflammatory medicines (both injected and oral) ease the symptoms.

Let's sum up on collagen: The good news is that it's very safe (after two allergy tests are given), provides a nice natural effect if injected correctly, and usually lasts three to six months. Also, if you don't like the way it looks, much of it will be gone or diminished in three to four months. The bad news is that, if you like collagen and it works well for you, it does have to be repeated anywhere from two to six times a year. Also, it's moderately expensive. (See Chapter 3 for more on collagen.)

Other filler agents. Fat transfers are an option for this area. Fat can be removed from one area of the body—for example, the hips or the inner thighs—and injected back into this area. The problem with both collagen and fat is that they're not permanent. Fat transfers may last longer than collagen, but their duration is very unpredictable. In some people, the fat will last only several months; in others, up to sev-

eral years. It isn't possible to predict prior to the fat transfer who will have a long-lasting result.

Also, fat transfers are performed with larger needles, so there's much more swelling and bruising than with collagen. You may need to stay home for one to two weeks after fat transfer—ask your dermatologist. As this procedure improves, more consistent effects and less downtime may be possible in the future.

Gortex grafts are also an option here. They're permanent but also have more downtime associated with their insertion. In addition, they can occasionally get infected, move, or be rejected by your body after placement.

Facial liposuction. If you have a very pronounced fold above the crease at the base of your nose, facial liposuction may help. In some people, the fat in the cheek area gradually shifts and collects at the nasolabial fold. A dermatologist experienced in facial liposuction may be able to reduce the fat there with excellent results.

Lip Lines

"I'm 35, but I used to smoke. Is it just my imagination, or are my upper lip lines quite a bit worse than my friends?"

It's probably not your imagination: Smoking does increase upper-lip lines due to the constant pursing of the lips to draw the smoke out of the cigarette. Plus, the smoke itself dries out the skin and deprives it of oxygen. Heavy smokers pay a significant price as they age as far as the wrinkling and yellowing of their skin is concerned.

We all get upper-lip lines as we get older. The movements of the mouth and lips when we eat, kiss, purse our lips, play musical instruments, put on makeup, smile, and talk all cause lines of expression to form as we age. And the gradual loss of the fatty layer (usually due to age) just under the skin makes the skin wrinkle. However, filler substances work quite well in this area.

Collagen is extremely versatile around the lips. Some patients want lips like Angelina Jolie, but most would like their lips to be just a little fuller than they are, or decrease the lines in that area. If you *do* decide you want fuller lips, go slowly and gradually so that you and your circle of friends aren't shocked (unless of course that's what you want). If you request just a little more at each visit, most people probably won't even notice that you've made a change.

Collagen fills upper-lip lines quite effectively. It's injected into the lines radiating up from the upper lip, where it fills up the wrinkle crease and smooths the skin out. Collagen can also be injected at the margins of the lips to pump up the lips and smooth the edges.

Using collagen on upper-lip lines or in the lips themselves can, in the hands of any practitioner, result in some lumpiness. Be sure to find an experienced dermatologist (or a nurse who *works* with one) before attempting to use collagen on this area. The lumpiness can last for months and be very annoying.

Sometimes your dermatologist might recommend that a tiny drop of Botox be injected into your upper lip if the muscle movement seems excessive. This has to be done carefully so that your lips move normally and symmetrically.

Laser resurfacing or TCA peels. These treatments work extremely well on upper-lip lines and are more permanent than collagen. However, you shouldn't get laser resurfacing or a TCA peel just around the mouth if you're sun damaged, for the peeled area will be the color and texture of new, fresh skin, while the rest of your face will remain unchanged. The areas won't match, and this variation in color and texture between the two parts of the face can look terrible. However, there are many different ways to prevent this. If you're sun damaged, the rest of your face needs to be peeled, too, even if it's a lighter peel to blend the areas.

A medium or deep TCA peel performed by an experienced dermatologist can be very effective for moderate upper-lip lines. Again, experience is the key to get the depth just right and to blend the area with the rest of the face.

Chin Dimpling

"As I've gotten older, I've developed funny little bumps and dimples in my chin that were never there before. What's causing these?"

If you look carefully, most people over the age of 40 have some dimpling—almost like a cobblestone appearance—in their chins. It becomes more pronounced in some of us than others.

The same culprits cause chin dimpling as many other lines on our faces: Sun damage reduces the elasticity in the support structure of the skin; loss of the fat pad in the chin causes some dimpling of the skin; and the action of the muscles of the chin and muscles pulling down at the corners of the mouth also aggravates this.

Again, filler agents, including collagen and fat in particular, work well here. The collagen or fat can be injected right into the dimpled area to lift it out. It's the same type of injection dermatologists use when treating depressed acne scars with collagen. If overactive muscles in this area are the problem, a small amount of Botox may be helpful. A more permanent solution is to have a plastic surgeon put in a chin implant—but this is usually overkill for a small number of dimples and probably isn't a realistic option unless you have a receding chin that has bothered you your entire life.

SUMMARY OF LINES OF FACIAL EXPRESSION: WHAT TO DO

The two most popular treatments to soften lines of facial expression—such as frown lines, crow's-feet, and forehead lines—are Botox and collagen. Botox injections relax the muscles under the skin so that the wrinkled skin also relaxes. Over time, the wrinkles may disappear as well. Collagen injections lift and fill lines of facial expression to make them less apparent.

- **Botox** works best for frown lines, crow's-feet around the eyes, horizontal forehead lines, and nasal scrunch lines.

- **Collagen** works best for plumping lips and filling upper-lip lines, and lines around the mouth and nose.

Injecting Botox and collagen is an art as well as a science. Be sure to find a dermatologist, physician's assistant, or nurse who's experienced and who listens to your concerns.

Laser resurfacing can also reduce the wrinkles of lines of expression, but you should consider it only if you also have deep wrinkles in your face in addition to prominent lines of expression. Let's take a look at those deep wrinkles in the next chapter.

ை ை ை   ை ை ை

3

DEEP
WRINKLES

The two previous chapters covered fine wrinkles and lines of expression. But what about those deeper furrows that come with age and sun exposure? Such creases can occur anywhere on the face—sometimes they're just the result of the gradual progression of lines of expression, such as deep frown or forehead lines; in other cases, fine wrinkles on the cheeks can deepen (with sun exposure or smoking) into pronounced grooves.

Deep wrinkles are more complicated than fine wrinkles and lines of expression because they have multiple causes. Each one of us will lose some elasticity in our skin as we age, and we'll also lose a bit of the fat pad underlying the skin that keeps it smooth and supple. But some of us have also had lots of sun exposure, which not only mottles and dries out the skin, but also damages its support structure. And then there are those of us who haven't eaten healthfully, or have smoked for many years—both of which take their toll over time.

What can we do about these deeper grooves? Is plastic surgery the answer? Can we smooth them out? Or are we stuck with them?

ର ର ର

WHAT ARE THE POSSIBLE CAUSES?

- Severe sun damage
- Age
- Smoking
- Weight changes
- Poor health

WHAT ARE THE POSSIBLE TREATMENTS?

- Sun protection
- CO_2 laser resurfacing
- Erbium laser resurfacing
- Noninvasive lasers
- Collagen
- Fat and other filler agents
- Botox
- Face-lift

POSSIBLE CAUSES

"I'm only 45 years old, but people often think I'm in my mid-50s. I do have a lot more wrinkles than most other women my age. Why?"

Since we're all individuals, there are a lot of different causes for this problem. The main factors are listed below.

Severe Sun Damage

Light from the sun, even through clouds, contains ultraviolet (UV) radiation, and ultraviolet radiation damages skin. I know that many of us grew up lusting after deep bronze tans, but too much sunlight is extremely harmful to the skin.

Have you ever noticed what happens to a leather or upholstered chair situated in front of a sunny window for a year or two? The colors in the fabric start to fade and discolor, and the leather gets stiff and hard compared to the areas not exposed to the sun. Ultimately, the leather cracks and the fabric starts to disintegrate. This is essentially what light and sunlight do to your skin over time.

Light—and not just direct sunlight—is responsible for many of the changes we see in our skin as we get older. It destroys elastic fibers and collagen in the skin, thins its outer barrier layer, and causes unsightly blood vessels and brown spots to appear.

Light from the sun has two main components that damage skin: UVB (sometimes called the "burning" ray) and UVA (light used in tanning booths). UVA rays used to be thought of as "safe" because they didn't usually cause sunburns—now we know that nothing could be further from the truth. Even though UVA rays may not always cause sunburns, they're just as responsible for skin cancers and blotchy, wrinkled skin. UVA radiation may, in fact, cause more damage because it's a longer wavelength of light than UVB. Thus, it penetrates more deeply into the skin, where it can damage the collagen and elastic fibers that support the skin and make it supple.

This is why, if you want to avoid more wrinkling and sun damage, you need to use a sunscreen that blocks *both UVA and UVB* every single morning on light-exposed areas. Most sunscreens block UVB, but many don't block UVA. Look for sunscreens that contain zinc or Parsol 1789/avobenzone, for they block UVA best. Sunscreens with titanium are also good. And remember, *tan* should be a four-letter word.

Outdoor occupations. There are a number of jobs that can predispose you to skin cancers and wrinkles, such as gardening, construction, forestry, ski instruction, or lifeguarding. But even truckers, pilots, couriers, and delivery people can be outside a lot, and they're also absorbing lots of UVA rays through window glass. Remember that *windows don't block UVA radiation.* Again, we almost always underestimate the amount of light and sun that we're getting, and it's important to protect ourselves with the measures mentioned above.

Outdoor sports. Outdoor activities, while wonderful for the body and mind, do carry increased risks for sun damage and skin cancers as well. And the extra ultraviolet light contributes to premature wrinkling.

Since I'm sure you don't want to live in a cave, you can prevent much of this damage with ample sun protection (including a hat). Look for sunscreens that are waterproof and sweatproof and contain at least a 4 to 7 percent concentration of zinc. A good one is the SkinCeuticals Sport Sunscreen with SPF 45, which is sold in dermatologists' offices or on the Internet. This one is expensive, so I recommend using it on high-risk areas, such as your head, neck, chest, hands, and forearms. You can then use the less expensive Coppertone Sport SPF 45 on the rest of your exposed areas.

Be sure to apply enough and reapply frequently. And be especially careful when skiing, hiking, or mountain climbing in high altitudes, or while participating in any water or snow sports.

A word about hats: You've got to *wear* them—they won't do you any good sitting in your car! And the best hat has a full brim, which is moderately wide and goes all the way around the hat. Of course, there are some sports for which full-brimmed hats just aren't practical, so if you're using a visor or a baseball cap, try to get one with a longer bill (a good one is the Patagonia spoonbill cap). Move the cap around a little to block the sun from different angles if you're running or hiking. You can also wear one of these under a bike helmet.

Golfers should take note that they're very much at risk for skin cancer. I've noticed over the years that many golfers don't consider themselves to be out in the sun all that much—consequently, many of them now have problems with skin cancer. If you play golf frequently, be sure to wear a hat with a full brim that extends all the way around (not just a visor), and apply sunscreen on all exposed areas. Protective clothing is even better if you're a serious golfer and spend a lot of time out on the links.

Five Ways to Save Your Skin Besides Sunscreen

1. Wear a hat. Try the Helen Kaminski hats (available at Nordstrom). They're straw, keep you cool, pack well, and wear like iron.
2. Stay under a shady tree or beach umbrella.
3. Swim or snorkel with an ultralight, sexy wetsuit.
4. Buy a Sun Precautions "big shirt" for walks in the sun on the beach—it's great over a bathing suit (visit **www.sunprecautions.com** to order one).
5. Swim early in the morning or late in the afternoon.

Age

Age has less to do with deep wrinkles than you might think. In an ideal world, we all would have stayed out of the sun or protected ourselves constantly while out in it, eaten well and exercised every day of our lives, and received state-of-the-art skin care. Sure, if we'd done all those things, we'd have very few wrinkles.

The reality is that I treat patients in their 50s, 60s, and 70s who have beautiful skin and look 10 to 20 years younger than their age. I also see women in their late 30s with lots of sun exposure whose skin is brown and blotchy, is significantly wrinkled, and has a dry and leathery texture.

I once saw a wonderful presentation that showed side-by-side photographs of an old Native American woman who had lived outdoors in the Southwest all of her life, and an elderly Buddhist monk who had spent almost all of his life indoors. The difference in the quality of their skin was really quite remarkable: The monk's skin was smooth, supple, and almost wrinkle free, but the face of the Native American woman was a leathery mass of deep wrinkles.

Smoking

Smoking not only poisons the lungs, it also poisons the circulation in the skin. You don't need to understand all the scientific details of smoking's effect on the body to see how bad it is for your skin. Just take a look at someone who has smoked for a while—you'll notice that their skin sags and is usually yellowish, wrinkled, and rough in texture.

Smoking deprives skin of the oxygen it needs to stay healthy and supple. The toxins that are in inhaled cigarette smoke also cause the blood vessels throughout the body to narrow, which in turn decreases blood flow to the skin. And the chemicals in cigarette smoke gradually destroy the small blood vessels in the skin itself.

Moreover, since smokers are constantly pursing their lips to drag the smoke out of the cigarette, they develop very deep upper- and lower-lip lines from the constant actions of the muscles underneath the skin.

Your skin and entire body will thank you if you can stop smoking. The first step is to talk to your family doctor about programs that are available to help you. As with alcohol, smoking can be very difficult to quit without a support group—there are just too many cues in daily life that are triggers for wanting a cigarette. Most smokers find that they have a number of these triggers, such as finishing a meal, lovemaking, stress, being around other smokers, and so on. Since smoking is so interwoven into life habits, it can be very difficult to quit without a doctor's help or the support of a group.

In addition to smoking-cessation programs, there are a number of medical aids that can help reduce nicotine cravings. Nicotine patches and gum can be extremely helpful as a way to get through the withdrawal period, and there are also a number of excellent books on the market that can inspire you and help you quit.

So, please talk to your doctor first. It's also beneficial to talk to people you know who have quit smoking to see what worked for them. Good luck!

Weight Changes

Fortunately, skin is very elastic, which is something that pregnant women are well aware of. When we're younger (and if we don't have a lot of sun damage), the skin has enough elasticity to contract back and forth to accommodate weight gains and losses fairly easily. As we get older and are more sun damaged, however, we lose some of that elasticity.

Patients sometimes ask whether weight loss will make them more wrinkled looking. The answer is: Sometimes. Some people have more elasticity in their skin than others. Pregnancy, for example, leaves some women with lots of stretch marks yet leaves others untouched. It's the same thing with weight loss: Some of us have skin that contracts quickly while others do it slowly or not at all.

It makes no sense to carry extra weight—and extra health risks—just to avoid the possibility of a few wrinkles. Plus, you should remember a couple of things: (1) Better nutrition, regular exercise, and a healthy lifestyle can do wonders for the appearance of your skin; and (2) much can be done nowadays to improve wrinkling. Better to lose the weight and improve your health and then tackle the wrinkles with some of the advances in modern dermatology.

Also keep in mind that skin contracts more slowly as we get older, so it's wise to wait for at least a year after losing a significant amount of weight to see how much the skin will contract on its own. Give your skin plenty of time to adjust to a new and slimmer you before spending time and money ridding yourself of wrinkles.

Poor Health

It's never too late to start taking care of your health in general. If you haven't been diligent about it in the past, just put all of that behind you and do your best from now on. If you're not sure how to start, ask your primary-care doctor and a good nutritionist to help you. While you don't need to eat salmon and brussels sprouts three times a day, good nutrition *is* important for healthy skin.

Remember that your skin gets assaulted every day: Sun and wind weather it, cuts and scrapes tear it, and normal disruptions such as pimples break its surface. Poor health and nutrition impair the skin's ability to repair itself from all of this wear and tear. The better your health, the faster your skin will heal itself. And the healthier your skin, the more it resists wrinkling.

POSSIBLE TREATMENTS

Sun Protection

It goes without saying that there's no point in treating existing wrinkles and sun-damaged skin without first making a commitment to prevent as much sun damage as possible in the future. Here are the key steps to take:

1. Apply a sunscreen with zinc or Parsol 1789/avobenzone *every day* on your face, neck, chest, hands, and forearms, or any other areas exposed regularly. Good sunscreens for daily use include M.D. Forté Environmental Protection Cream SPF 30, SkinCeuticals Daily Sun Defense SPF 20 or Ultimate UV Defense SPF 30, Cetaphil Daily Facial Moisturizer SPF 15, or Clinique City Block SPF 15.

2. Wear a waterproof, sweatproof sunscreen, SPF 30 or higher, when involved in outdoor athletics, hiking, or swimming. Reapply often. A good one is SkinCeuticals Sport SPF 45. Coppertone Sport SPF 45 is less expensive but doesn't have zinc in it.

3. Wear a hat when out in the direct sun. Protective clothing is better than sunscreen. A company called Sun Precautions makes good sun-protective clothing, and they market their clothes through stores, a catalog, and via the Internet (**www.sunprecautions.com**).

CO_2 Laser Resurfacing

"I'm 65 and am good about sun protection now, but I really wasn't in the past. I have a lot of deep wrinkling throughout my entire cheek area and around my eyes and mouth. What are my options for fixing this?"

If you have a lot of deep wrinkles that aren't just confined to the areas around the eye and the mouth, CO_2 laser resurfacing is still the best and most permanent option other than a face-lift. This laser uses a concentrated beam of light to completely remove the top layer of skin in a very precise and controlled way, which allows you to grow back a top layer of new skin that's fresh and not sun damaged.

The depth of the laser peel can be customized just for you, so if you have more wrinkles around your mouth, for example, more laser passes can be done there, and so on. This type of laser resurfacing is sometimes referred to as a *nonsurgical face-lift*. Here are the advantages:

— CO_2 laser resurfacing provides noticeable collagen tightening, lifting the skin a bit and thereby providing a sharper jawline and less drooping on the face overall.

— Fresh new "baby skin" will grow in after the resurfacing, so there are major improvements in texture and color.

— The process "resurfaces" right over the wrinkles, removing almost all of the fine wrinkles and most of the medium-depth wrinkles; it reduces the deeper ones as well.

If the resurfacing is done correctly, you can usually expect about a 40 to 60 percent reduction in wrinkles; some people get significantly more than that, even up to 70 or 80 percent in certain cases.

Your own expectations are very important in laser resurfacing. If you expect all your wrinkles to disappear, you'll be disappointed. But laser resurfacing *can* make a significant improvement in the appearance of your skin. Here are the main disadvantages:

— You may experience a tough first week post-procedure. It takes a full week for that new baby skin to grow back in, and there's a lot of swelling and oozing in the initial four days.

— There's a long recovery time. It can be a full two weeks before you'll want to go out of the house, and then your skin will be pink to red, and sensitive for an average of one to three months. This redness will occasionally last up to six months.

— There's more potential for complications because of the depth of the peel and the fact the skin is "open" and vulnerable to infections. Rare scarring does occur, and some resurfaced areas can end up looking whiter than others.

CO_2 laser resurfacing shouldn't be taken lightly. It requires a significant commitment of your time and money and has risks associated with it, so it's extremely important to find a dermatologist who's experienced in this procedure before undertaking it. In my opinion, the risks are very manageable as long as the dermatologist and/or nurses involved are skilled and caring.

Unfortunately, CO_2 resurfacing has received some bad press because it's been used by physicians who weren't qualified or who didn't adequately educate their patients about the post-procedure period. This difficult first post-op week can be made more comfortable for you with the right dressings, medications, and support from your doctor and nurse. It doesn't have to be a lonely, difficult experience.

CO_2 resurfacing does require anesthesia. I've found that the best option is to have a board-certified anesthesiologist present for the entire procedure (and most of the recovery period) to provide what's known as *conscious sedation*. This is intravenous sedation that allows you to remain comfortable, pain free, and very sleepy during the procedure.

Some dermatologists will use regional blocks by injecting an anesthetic agent into the nerves that go to certain areas of the face. (In fact, your dentist may have used this method for certain kinds of dental surgery.) This is usually augmented with local anesthesia, which is injected directly into the skin. This combination of regional blocks with local anesthesia works reasonably well, but you have to endure the discomfort of the injections. Again, it's best if a board-certified anesthesiologist can be present throughout the procedure to provide some intravenous sedation for comfort and pain control.

Erbium Laser Resurfacing

If you have mild to moderate wrinkling, erbium laser resurfacing may be a better choice for you than CO_2 resurfacing. The erbium laser works like the CO_2 laser, but it takes off even thinner layers of skin, enabling the surgeon to be very precise in the depth of the peel.

The erbium laser is ideal for areas where the skin is particularly thin, such as around the eyes or on the neck. Recovery is faster and the complications are fewer than with CO_2 lasers because the procedure isn't as deep. The other advantage to erbium resurfacing is that it causes less post-procedure redness than CO_2 resurfacing.

Some dermatologists use this process for resurfacing deeper wrinkles. This can work, but it requires many more passes with the laser handpiece than with CO_2 resurfacing.

Noninvasive Lasers

This is an evolving area. These lasers don't break the skin—instead, they heat or stimulate the cells deep in the skin to make more collagen. There's some evidence now that these lasers are helpful for fine wrinkles and maybe even moderate wrinkles. However, at this point in time, they don't do a particularly good job with deep wrinkles. As more research is done, that assessment may change.

Collagen

"What's collagen used for? How do I know if I'd be a good candidate for it?"

A good candidate has lines primarily around the nose and mouth. Collagen can fill in the area at the base of the nose; the corners of the mouth; the lips and upper- and lower-lip lines; and smaller lines and dimples around the chin and lower cheeks. It can also be used to fill in scars.

Although collagen can be used around crow's-feet, it's sometimes lumpy. Botox is usually better for frown lines, crow's-feet, horizontal forehead lines, and other lines of facial expression, for it will relax those muscles and soften the wrinkles that result from the contraction of those muscles.

Collagen can become prohibitively expensive if you have deep lines all over your face. At that point, you might want to consider laser resurfacing or a face-lift.

"What is collagen?"

It's a natural protein that provides structural support for human tissue. Collagen occurs throughout the body—in skin, muscle, tendon, and bone. Even some heart valves used during surgery are made of it.

The collagen in human skin is very similar to that found in certain animals. Injectable collagen, such as Zyderm and Zyplast, is made of collagen from cow skin that has been highly purified.

"How is it made?"

Collagen made by the McGhan Medical Corp. is taken from cows grazed in a single closed herd from one ranch in Northern California. The herd is carefully managed, isn't fed any animal products, and is also frequently tested for disease. The collagen is then highly purified and sterilized in laboratories that conform to the highest standards.

"How much will collagen improve my wrinkles or lips?"

That depends on your goals and your budget. Again, if you expect perfection, you're going to be disappointed, but if you're a good candidate for collagen, you can expect 50 to 90 percent correction depending on the location and depth of the wrinkles and the skill of the provider.

Collagen injection is as much an art as it is a science. Expect a "learning curve" with you and your doctor—it usually takes one to three sessions for you to see how it looks so that you can let your doctor know where you'd like more or less.

"How long does it last?"

Most of the time, you can expect collagen to last three to six months. The first two treatments are often performed approximately two weeks apart and build up a base of collagen. After that, the number of treatments depends on you and your goals, but treatments every three to six months are most common to maintain the collagen. Areas that move a lot, such as the lips, tend to wear off sooner than areas that are a little "quieter," such as the cheeks and around the chin. In a few unlucky individuals, collagen is absorbed faster and may only last two months.

"How much does collagen generally cost?"

This depends completely on the number of syringes needed and what city you live in, but the treatments generally range from $300 to $1,000.

"How is collagen injected?"

It comes in syringes manufactured by McGhn Medical and is usually injected with tiny needles comparable in size to those used for acupuncture treatments.

Collagen is a soft substance; when warmed to room temperature, it's about the consistency of thick custard. Usually the skin is numbed with a topical numbing cream such as lidocaine. When collagen is injected, the skin numbs even more because the collagen itself has a small amount of lidocaine added to it.

"Do the injections hurt?"

To ease your apprehension, a good dermatologist or nurse will talk to you at some length before making any injections. You may find that the injections are somewhat uncomfortable, particularly around the nose or lips. However, the lidocaine in the collagen can help numb the area temporarily.

Many patients report that discomfort with the first injections decreases with further injections. There are now also several lidocaine preparations in cream form—one of the most popular is called ELA-Max. It's rubbed into the skin approximately 45 minutes and then 20 minutes before the collagen injections and helps to decrease the discomfort.

"Are there any side effects?"

Yes, but they're usually negligible. Minor stinging, bruising, and temporary swelling are common. Bruising generally resolves itself within three to ten days, and swelling may last a few hours to a day or two. Makeup can often be applied right after the injections.

Very rare complications are scabs or blisters that can result in small scars, and flulike symptoms in less than 5 in 1,000 treatments. Also, injections can occasionally provoke an outbreak of cold sores (facial herpes simplex). Even if collagen treatments are successful, the rare patient may complain of depression or emotional difficulties. Also, collagen does cause alergic reactions in rare instances.

"How do I know if I'm allergic to it?"

Your doctor will test you before you begin the process. Skin testing for collagen allergies is done in the forearm, much like a TB test. A tiny amount of collagen is placed in the skin in that area. The site is then watched for about one month to make sure there's no redness, swelling, or itching. If, after one month, the site of the first collagen test is normal, then a second test is done, usually in the other forearm. If either of the skin-test sites show any reaction, then collagen treatment shouldn't be undertaken. This is extremely important, since experiencing an allergic reaction to a substance in your face can be very unpleasant.

A rare type of allergic reaction to collagen occurs in about one to five percent of those tested, even though they may have had two negative tests. This very unusual occurrence is called a *delayed hypersensitivity reaction.* The reaction may consist of prolonged swelling, redness, itching, or firmness at some or all of the injection sites.

If you're that unlucky individual in a hundred who gets a delayed hypersensitivity reaction, it will generally last between three and six months. In some very rare cases, the reaction has lasted for more than a year. Some of the symptoms can be alleviated by injecting anti-inflammatory medicine into the irritated sites, or, in some cases, using various *oral* anti-inflammatory medications. Again, the good news is that even if this does happen, it's rare and almost always goes away.

"Who shouldn't have collagen treatments?"

If you're absolutely terrified of needles, please do yourself a favor and don't undertake collagen injections. Check with your doctor first if you're pregnant (why take any risks?), have problems with clotting, or have diseases such as lupus or scleroderma.

I'm also of the opinion that highly stressful times in life aren't a good time to begin collagen treatments. And if you're depressed, it's best to wait until you're feeling better to begin.

"Is there anything I should avoid doing before my first collagen treatment?"

Yes, be sure to reread your dermatologist's written instructions. (If you've lost them, call and have them sent to you.)

Many doctors will ask you to avoid anything that will increase your chances of bruising for a week before your treatment, which may include aspirin, ibuprofen, naproxen, and extra vitamin E. If you're taking any of these substances for medical reasons, check with your primary-care doctor before you stop taking them.

Collagen Dos and Don'ts

- **Do** purchase some lidocaine cream to use about 45 minutes and then about 20 minutes before your treatment to make you more comfortable.
- **Don't** take aspirin, ibuprofen, or naproxen for a week prior to your treatment because you'll be more likely to bruise.
- **Do** make firm decisions before your treatment as to which areas on your face you want to try to correct.
- **Don't** schedule your treatment right before an important social engagement, since you may be puffy and red for about 24 hours.

Fat Transfer

"I've heard that using my own fat to fill in wrinkles is better because it's more natural."

As we age, we lose the soft layer of fat just under the skin. For most areas of the body, this loss has little effect on appearance; but the gradual loss of fat (in addition to sun damage, age, and so on) on the face makes the skin appear more wrinkled.

Many years ago, researchers had the bright idea of taking fat from parts of the body that have too much and putting it into parts of the face that don't have enough. In most cases, fat is removed from an area on the inner thigh, buttocks, hips, or abdomen. It's washed and then reinjected into the face. Sometimes the fat can be kept frozen for months if multiple injections are needed.

The advantage, of course, to using one's own fat is that there isn't any possibility of an allergic reaction. It's a completely "natural" substance that can be transferred with a syringe. Fat transfer is a highly promising treatment, and research in this area is very active. But results aren't predictable yet.

One problem with fat transfer is getting the fat cells to live ("take") in their new site. Sometimes they die relatively quickly and are carried off by the body's own mechanism for getting rid of dead cells. In this situation, the fat transfer does not last any longer than collagen does. As of this writing, the amount of time fat lasts is very unpredictable from person to person, which makes it difficult to give an accurate estimate of how often it will need to be repeated.

The other disadvantage with fat transfer is that a larger needle needs to be used compared to those used with collagen injections. These larger needles cause significantly more bruising and swelling and, consequently, more patient downtime. After collagen injections, you can usually go right back to work and other activities, but fat transfers may cause enough bruising to keep you home for a week or more.

Techniques for fat transfer have been improving steadily over the past five years. This is an area to watch closely as results become more reliable.

Other Filler Agents

Collagen is the most widely used filler agent and has a long track record. It's very safe as long as you're not allergic to it. Below are some of the alternatives to collagen, with their advantages and disadvantages explained.

Keep in mind that this is an area of active research. Some filler agents have been used for years in Europe, Canada, and South America but haven't been approved in the U.S. by the Food and Drug Administration (FDA) as yet. Some of these agents are currently in the pipeline, but the FDA has the toughest standards in the world for drugs and medications, so approval can take several years. This is generally a good thing for consumer safety, but the waiting time can sometimes be frustrating.

Hyaluronic acid. This hasn't been approved by the FDA yet, nor is it even available in the United States, but reports indicate that it's coming in the next few years. Hyaluronic acid is a substance found naturally in the deeper layer of the skin, called the *dermis*. There are three forms of it: Hylaform—which is made from rooster combs; and Restylane and Perlane—which have been used extensively in Europe, are made in a laboratory, and do not come from an animal source.

Like collagen, hyaluronic acid can be moderately uncomfortable, but topical numbing creams tend to ease the discomfort. Following are its **advantages:**

- At present, this procedure does not require allergy testing, although a few cases of allergic reactions have now been recorded in medical literature.

- Its safety profile may be better than collagen.
- The procedure causes very little bruising or downtime.
- It may be slightly better for the lips because it retains water better than collagen.
- The discomfort and cost factors are about the same as that of collagen.

Disadvantages:

- This procedure hasn't been approved by the FDA for cosmetic use yet, and it's currently unavailable in the United States.
- It's slightly more difficult for doctors to inject correctly than collagen.
- Occasional temporary lumps do occur.
- Longevity appears to be about the same as collagen: approximately two to six months depending on the person, the area injected, and the type of hyaluronic acid used.

Autologen. This is your own collagen. It's manufactured by sending large pieces of skin (generated during plastic surgery) to a manufacturer, who then extracts your own collagen and puts it back into syringes under carefully controlled laboratory conditions. Its advantage is that there's no risk of allergic reaction, and no risk of any viral infection you didn't already have.

The disadvantage is that it needs to be scheduled with a plastic surgeon, which makes it very impractical for most people and very expensive. But if you're having plastic surgery anyway, you may want to talk to your surgeon about this.

Botox

Botox is really the best choice for lines of expression such as frown lines, forehead lines, or crow's-feet, because it acts to relax the muscle under the skin. When the muscle doesn't move the skin, the skin doesn't wrinkle. Botox stops the skin from wrinkling, and many wrinkles will disappear completely over time.

To stop deep wrinkles from continuing to furrow, Botox is most useful around the eyes, on the forehead, on the frown lines in the center of the forehead, and (in certain special cases) in very small amounts for lines around the mouth. It can also be useful in and around the neck for certain types of wrinkles. It can't be used at all for wrinkles in the cheek area or for those around the mouth (most of the time).

Face-Lift

The proper surgical name for a face-lift is *rhytidectomy,* which literally means "to surgically remove wrinkles." Face-lifts should be performed by a board-certified plastic surgeon—preferably one in your own community who's been recommended to you by both physicians and friends. This isn't an area where you should try to save money. This is your *face,* and the potential for permanent complications from surgery is significant.

Consider a face-lift an option if you have a loss of elasticity with excess skin hanging down around the jawline, chin, and neck (sometimes referred to as *jowls*). A small amount of fat under the chin, a little wrinkling through the cheek area, or loss of contour through the jawline can usually be corrected quite nicely with other modalities, such as CO_2 laser resurfacing or the much less invasive liposuction (done under the chin with a very small needle). But if you really do have a lot of lax skin and wrinkles around the jawline and under the chin, a face-lift may be your best option.

Remember, however, that a face-lift doesn't do anything to improve the texture and color of your skin, nor will it address lines around the lips, so some kind of peel or laser resurfacing around the mouth may also be needed.

Also, procedures such as eyelid surgery *(blepharoplasty)* don't generally correct the small, crepelike wrinkles under the eye. You may need peels, gentle laser photorejuvenation, or CO_2 or erbium laser resurfacing for that area if texture or color is a problem. Good plastic surgeons will give you an accurate assessment of the improvements you can expect.

SUMMARY OF DEEP WRINKLES: WHAT TO DO

With deep wrinkles, an ounce of prevention is worth a pound of cure. And most of this prevention should be devoted to sun protection, for the majority of the wrinkling stems from sun damage. Unfortunately, many individuals in our society still prize the tanned look. A tan used to be a sign of wealth, a status symbol for those who could take vacations to sunny climates. But we pay the price for all that sun exposure: wrinkles, blotchiness, and leathery skin in our 50s and beyond.

If you start applying the following measures at a young age, your skin may stay smooth for many years:

- Use a good-quality **sunscreen** with zinc or Parsol 1789/ avobenzone every day.
- Wear **hats** and sun-protective clothing.

- Eat a **balanced, nutritious diet** and **exercise** regularly.
- **Avoid smoking** and engaging in other poor health habits.
- Take a **multivitamin** daily.

If, however, your skin has deep wrinkles, the nonsurgical options for treating them are:

- **Laser resurfacing** costs between $4,000 and $7,000 and entails considerable downtime, but it can tighten the skin and significantly reduce wrinkles on the face. Much lighter laser peels can be done on the neck and chest.
- **Collagen and other filler agents** can fill out and reduce specific wrinkles very nicely; the cost makes it best for a limited

number of deep wrinkles, usually around the mouth and nose.

Since lasers can treat both deep wrinkles and fine wrinkles, and because lasers are a relatively new development, the next chapter provides a detailed explanation of lasers: how they work, what a treatment is like, and how to find a competent laser dermatologist.

ೲ ೲ ೲ   ೲ ೲ ೲ

4

LASERS

Lasers can now do so much to improve your skin that they have changed the landscape of cosmetic dermatology. They can remove redness and treat rosacea; help with fine wrinkles with almost no downtime; eliminate brown spots and age spots; reduce or get rid of unwanted hair; dramatically improve deeper wrinkles, acne scars, and texture problems; and can even eliminate certain leg veins.

Earlier chapters covered some of these topics in connection with particular skin issues. But this chapter will provide you with a summary of lasers and will help you find a good dermatologic laser surgeon, evaluate a laser center, choose an appropriate laser treatment for your problem, and help you avoid costly mistakes.

FINDING A GOOD DOCTOR

- Other doctors' referrals
- Physician credentials
- Recommendations from family and friends
- Advertising
- Types of laser centers
- Laser costs

YOUR LASER EXPERIENCE

- Making an appointment
- Your consultation
- The treatment itself
- The healing phase
- Treatments in series
- Long-term expectations

DIFFERENT LASER SYSTEMS

- For redness
- For age spots and brown spots
- For hair removal and maintenance
- For sun damage
- For leg veins
- For deep wrinkles and acne scars

FINDING A GOOD DOCTOR

Other Doctors' Referrals

"How can I find a good laser surgeon?"

If you have a great doctor in another specialty, such as internal medicine, family practice, or gynecology, he or she will often know who the other excellent doctors in town are. So this is the best place to start when seeking a referral to a dermatologist and a laser center.

If you haven't been to a doctor in a long time, this is a great opportunity to go. Schedule your annual physical, and at the end of the appointment, ask about referrals (try to get several names so that you'll be able to compare doctors). Be sure to tell your physician that you're interested in cosmetic or laser work, since some dermatologists still only do medical dermatology.

Once you get the name of several dermatologists with laser centers, call and make an appointment. Most dermatologists have special times available for cosmetic work and consultations, so if you're primarily interested in laser work, ask for a laser consultation—you may be seen faster. But be prepared to wait several months for a medical dermatology appointment. Most good dermatologists are booked anywhere from four to twelve weeks in advance. If you prefer to get to know your doctor while having your moles checked, acne treated, or other medical problems attended to, that's fine—just be aware that most dermatologists are busy, and they may not be able to spend a lot of time on your cosmetic concerns at that visit. You may want to make a cosmetic appointment to discuss those particular issues.

Physician Credentials

"I asked my dermatologist about her credentials and training, but I really didn't understand what she said."

Even though many books explaining how to find a good doctor suggest inquiring about credentials, most patients have a difficult time evaluating them. For instance, you probably won't really know which residency programs are the outstanding ones, whether the doctor graduated with honors in medical school, or whether she was one of the top trainees in her residency program.

Some dermatologists now have Websites where they post their credentials. Look for honors such as Alpha Omega Alpha, which is the honor society in medical school, and any national awards or grants. A faculty affiliation with a university, however, isn't always what it seems. Some doctors will list a clinical faculty appointment (such as "Associate Clinical Professor"), which is often given to practicing doctors who volunteer a small amount of time to teach residents each year. The appointment doesn't necessarily mean that the doctor conducts any research or is otherwise connected with the university. "Clinical" professors at most universities usually aren't on the full- or part-time faculty.

As far as residency programs go, you can't assume that a state residency program is less prestigious than a private university program. For example, some large state university training programs are actually ranked higher than some Ivy League training programs.

Laser education is even more difficult to evaluate because most dermatologic laser surgeons didn't receive their laser training in their residency program—they got it in post-residency courses, preceptorships, and workshops. This is gradually changing as more residency programs begin to adopt additional formal laser training requirements.

Other physicians are probably the most helpful in evaluating another doctor's credentials. They'll usually know who's well trained and who isn't.

Recommendations from Family and Friends

"My mother raves about her dermatologist. Should I assume he'll be right for me, too?"

Referrals from family and friends are a little bit tricky. Many people have trouble evaluating a doctor's expertise, so they make their recommendations based upon whether or not they like the doctor. While bedside manner is certainly important, it doesn't necessarily mean that you'll be getting the highest quality work. The best referral is from a friend or family member whose skin you've seen improve noticeably over a period of months or even years under the care of the doctor to whom they're referring you. If the dermatologist is getting great results with your loved ones, and you can see the improvement yourself, that's a pretty good recommendation. Don't forget to ask for referrals from friends, family members, or neighbors who are doctors or nurses themselves.

Advertising

"If a laser center advertises in my local newspaper, doesn't that mean they're reputable?"

Not necessarily. Even though there's been a marked increase in the last five or ten years in physician advertising in newspapers and weekly magazines, on the radio, and sometimes even on television, I ask this question: If these physicians are really top-notch and are already booked with appointments, why do they need to advertise? The fact that a physician or laser center is advertising means that they need more business. Why aren't they busy enough? Most of the top dermatologists and laser centers don't need to advertise, since they already have more than enough patients.

Be particularly skeptical about clinics or centers that just advertise one type of procedure (for example, hair removal). Some of these places aren't supervised or even owned by physicians. Many claim that they're physician supervised but, in fact, the doctor isn't actually on the premises or is only there rarely. The nursing staff operating the lasers is often only minimally experienced. In addition, some of these clinics have taken large fees in advance and have then gone bankrupt, leaving the patients empty-handed. Look for physicians and laser centers that have been well established in the area for at least three to five years before committing any large amounts of money.

The yellow pages. Looking in the yellow pages is unreliable. Unfortunately, the size of the ad has absolutely nothing to do with the quality of the dermatologist. In fact, in some cities there seems to be an inverse relationship between the size of the ads and the quality of the practice. Some excellent physicians, in fact, have taken their listings out of the yellow pages (except for their addresses). It's been my experience that when doctors are really busy, they don't need to spend money on advertising.

Is Your Dermatologist Really a Dermatologist?

Believe it or not, once a doctor graduates from medical school and does an internship, she can legally call herself anything she wants. A family practitioner or someone board certified in urology can decide that she wants to call herself a dermatologist and hang out a shingle, even though she has no speciality training in dermatology at all. In my opinion, this is unethical, but it *is* unfortunately legal. Here's how to make sure your dermatologist is for real:

1. Check the Website of the American Academy of Dermatology (**www.aad.org**), which has a list of all the board-certified dermatologists in the country by state and by name. (The site also has a lot of other useful information.)

2. Don't ask your doctor if she's board certified. She may say yes because she's board certified in *urology*. Instead, ask, "Are you board certified in dermatology?"

3. Check the directory of your local county medical society. Since doctors have to verify their credentials to join such societies, the listing will usually contain accurate information about board certification.

Types of Laser Centers

"Our area has several different laser centers. How do I figure out which one is best?"

There are many different types of laser centers now. Some small centers can provide a very high level of service, while some larger centers may be less personal. The critical factor isn't size, it's caliber of care.

Look for a center associated with a well-known dermatologist who devotes a significant amount of time to laser work. The physicians should be on-site most of the time to supervise any nonphysician personnel such as registered nurses or certified physician assistants. You can also ask the dermatologist or the laser center staff about credentials and laser education.

Avoid places where the laser service doesn't seem like a good fit, such as an ophthalmologist adding a laser for hair removal or a family practitioner adding a laser to treat leg veins. In general, the quality of care will be better in a dermatologist's office that has a significant amount of time dedicated to laser work.

Laser Costs

"I've been calling around to different offices to compare prices, and one of them is significantly less expensive than the others. Should I go there?"

This is an area, like plastic surgery, where shopping for bargain-basement prices isn't a great idea. The best dermatologic laser surgeons will usually charge somewhere from the median to the higher end of the cost spectrum because they're better, and are usually busy. They also often have a greater variety of laser equipment—since such equipment is very expensive, this will usually drive the cost up a bit as well. Also, excellent laser physicians tend to have excellent staff that they treat respectfully and pay well. Keep in mind that while the quality of the physician you choose is highly important, the caliber of the team working with that physician is crucial, too, so you should find a high-quality laser center *and* a good dermatologic laser practitioner.

Laser costs do vary a lot by geographical area: A laser center in New York City will charge substantially more than one in Omaha, reflecting the difference in the cost of doing business in those two areas. However, larger urban areas may be the only places in your state where you can find an excellent laser surgeon. Many small towns just don't have the population mass to support a laser center.

৩৩ ৩৩ ৩৩

———————————————— ◇ ————————————————

How Is a Dermatologist Trained?

A dermatologist is a specialist trained specifically in the care of skin, hair, and nails, including diagnosis and treatment of skin diseases and skin cancers (including surgery); dermatopathology; and the promotion of skin health.

A dermatologist must complete four years of college and four years of medical school (like all doctors). Then comes an internship, and in many cases a residency in internal medicine or pediatrics, for a total of three more years. (In my case, I did a residency in internal medicine and am board certified in that as well.) Then comes three years of specialized dermatology residency. By the end of all that, a dermatologist will have eight to ten years of medical education *in addition to* a basic college degree.

———————————————— ◇ ————————————————

YOUR LASER EXPERIENCE

Making an Appointment

"I think I'm ready to do something about my sun-damaged skin. What should I ask the doctor's receptionist?"

Okay, you've finally decided that you're ready. You have the names of several doctors, so you pick up that phone to make your first call. But let's suppose that you're put on hold for a long time or you reach someone who's a real grump . . . don't give up on that office just yet. Excellent doctors will usually have wonderful staff and systems set up to help you feel welcome, but not always. And anyone who has ever worked at a front desk knows that there are occasional off days when the volume of calls is high, or certain patients are requiring extra time. My advice would be to hang up courteously and then try again the next day. If you try twice or even three times and get the same treatment, it's probably best to scratch that office off your list.

Schedule a cosmetic consultation. When you do reach an office that appeals to you, schedule a cosmetic consultation. Be sure to let the receptionist know what treatments you're interested in; for example, if you know you're interested in Botox treatments, just say so. If you're not sure, say that you're interested in repairing sun damage or seeing what you can do about wrinkles. There will often be a charge (ranging anywhere from $50 to $250) for this consultation, but sometimes the fee can be applied to your first treatment.

Some offices have different consultants for different problems. There may be one nurse who does consultations for Botox and collagen, while another handles all of the laser consultations. You'll usually be seen by a nurse who specializes in that area, or by the doctor herself. Often, if the nurse spends time with you for the majority of the consultation, the physician will come in at the end to answer any final questions you might have.

Make a medical appointment. You can also call and make a medical appointment with a dermatologist, especially if you need treatment for acne or rosacea, or if you need to have your moles checked anyway. Just be aware that there may be a wait of several months for a good dermatologist, and that this isn't the appointment to get into an in-depth discussion of your cosmetic issues. After your dermatologist has attended to your medical problems, *then* you can mention your concerns; at that point, your doctor will often give you some preliminary information to begin reading and set up a cosmetic consultation.

Legally and ethically, dermatologists must strictly separate their medical and cosmetic work. Medical dermatology is usually covered by insurance, but cosmetic dermatology isn't. Medical appointments will be billed to your insurance company, but *you* will need to pay for appointments for cosmetic concerns or treatments yourself, at the time services are rendered. Insurance companies will not and should not pay for cosmetic services. *Never* ask a doctor to bill a cosmetic service to your insurance company—this is insurance fraud, which is a felony with steep fines attached to it. An excellent dermatologist would never knowingly or willingly commit fraud.

Your Consultation

"I have a cosmetic consultation set up with my doctor and her laser nurse in two weeks. What should I bring with me? And what should I ask?"

Getting there. Most offices will call you to confirm the consultation time a day or two before. If they don't, then it's wise to call and confirm the appointment yourself to make sure that everything is correct. It also helps to locate the address the night before and make sure that you know exactly how to get there. If you've never been to that office before, leave extra time so you're not late. You may also want to arrive 10 to 15 minutes early so that the office staff can make up a chart for you and you'll have time to fill out paperwork.

Since all doctors' offices run on a time schedule, if you're late you may be asked to reschedule so as to not inconvenience other patients. If you're stuck in a horrible traffic jam and have a cell phone, be sure to call the office immediately, give them a time frame, and ask if you should still come. Most well-run offices run on time, or no more than 30 minutes behind schedule. (And, when you do arrive at your appointment, it's perfectly reasonable to ask the front desk if the doctor tends to be on time or not.)

Bring a list. It's worthwhile to prepare a list of your concerns and bring them to your appointment.

This will help the cosmetic nurse specialist and your dermatologist answer all of your questions. Your consultation is really an opportunity to get to know the doctor and her staff and understand all of the options available to treat you. You may be given printed material such as pamphlets, and even your consent forms may contain valuable information. You might be asked to watch short videos regarding the procedures you're interested in.

Look for a warm, individual approach—not a cookie-cutter format. The nurse and doctor should not only give you the basic information they need to transmit, but they should also answer questions and concerns that you may have. The consultation should cover:

- information about how this particular treatment will help you achieve your goals;

- a detailed account of how the treatment is done, and approximately how many treatments will be needed;

- any preparations you'll need to make prior to the treatment;

- what to expect during the treatment (including any possible complications);

- what type of care you'll need after the procedure and if there are any restrictions on your activities;

- a brief review of your basic skin-care program to make sure that it includes good-quality sunscreen and renewal products at night; and

- the expected costs of the procedure.

After the consultation, the nurse will probably dictate a summary for you. You should also be given her phone number so that if you have any questions after you've reviewed the written material or consultation letter, you can call someone who has in-depth knowledge.

It isn't a good idea to ask the reception staff detailed medical information, since they're not doctors or nurses and usually don't have the authorization to answer specific medical questions.

The Treatment Itself

"My first laser treatment is next week. Is there anything I should do to get ready?"

Before your first treatment. One week prior to your first treatment, be sure to review all of the printed information that you've been given about the procedure. It may contain certain things that you need to do, such as avoiding aspirin or ibuprofen for one week prior to the procedure.

This literature may also contain information about items you need to bring with you that day, such as support hose for leg-vein laser treatments. And you may need to adjust your workout schedule to accommodate the treatment. For example, you shouldn't do yoga for 24 hours after Botox treatments, since many yoga positions are performed upside down and might cause the Botox to migrate.

After you've reviewed your written information, if you have any important questions that might affect the scheduling of the appointment, call the office right away. Many offices have a one- to two-week cancellation policy for cosmetic procedures—if you cancel too late, you may be billed in full for the procedure. Most questions, however, can wait until the time of your initial appointment.

During your first treatment, you'll usually be asked to sign a consent form if you haven't done so already. Photographs will often be taken, which will be kept in your chart and are for the use of the doctor and nurse only. However, if you have any concerns about them being published, be sure to voice them.

During the treatment. You should be made as comfortable as possible. You may have been asked to apply a topical "numbing" cream that usually has 4 or 5 percent lidocaine in it. It works best if applied 30 to 45 minutes before and then 15 minutes before the treatment. And after you're put in the treatment room, more lidocaine may be applied before the treatment begins.

Many cosmetic and laser centers have soothing music and blankets available if you're cold. If you're uncomfortable for any reason, be sure to let your physician's assistant, nurse, or doctor know. The duration of the treatments themselves varies depending on what's being done. For example, a short spot treatment might take 15 minutes, while a hair-removal treatment on the legs might take an hour and a half.

Ask how long the treatments will take *before* you arrive so you can plan your next appointment accordingly. It's usually a good idea to give yourself at least an hour before your next appointment so that you have plenty of time if the treatment runs just a little bit over or if you need to spend time applying makeup afterwards.

"I'm scared that the laser treatment will be painful."

Laser treatments usually feel like a very mild rubber-band snap on the face, and most patients tolerate them fairly easily. Again, numbing cream prior to this procedure will help. There's sometimes mild to moderate swelling associated with laser treatments—cool ice packs may be applied immediately after the procedure to reduce it.

Possible bruising. Many dermatologists will ask you to try to avoid certain substances that make you slightly more likely to bruise, such as aspirin, ibuprofen, or naproxen; vitamin E; alcoholic beverages the night before; or herbs such as St. John's wort or Ginkgo biloba.

But don't worry if you've forgotten—it won't affect how well the treatment works. Laser treatments can be done very safely even if you've taken one of the above, so don't cancel the appointment if you've taken an Advil—your chance of a bruise is just a little higher. If you're not sure if you've messed up the entire procedure, call the nurse to ask. Most of the time you'll be told to keep your appointment, and special measures may be taken to help you avoid any bruising. Some of us are just naturally prone to bruising, and any cosmetic treatment can cause it, no matter how gentle the technique. It's helpful to come prepared for small bruises:

Bring your favorite concealer, powder, and foundation with you.

Makeup. Many dermatologists will allow you to apply makeup right after a laser procedure, as long as there are no breaks in the skin. One nice item is a cover-up pencil, which is available at the Prescriptives counter at many department stores. This has two sides to it: One side has an apricot color that covers purplish discoloration very well; the other side has a tone that matches your skin color. Use the apricot side first and then apply the concealer over it—you'll get quite nice coverage. (Dermablend's products also work well: **www.dermablend.com**.)

Payment. Be sure to find out which payment methods the office accepts. Most cosmetic dermatology and laser centers accept a wide range of payment methods, but it doesn't hurt to check first.

The Healing Phase

"Will my dermatologist give me instructions telling me what to do after the laser treatment?"

Yes. Written instructions for care after your procedure will usually be found either in your consent form or given to you as a separate sheet of instructions immediately after the procedure. Dermatologists vary as far as what they may have you do—be sure to check with your own doctor for her specific recommendations.

There are some general post-procedure principles that apply to most laser treatments: Do only very gentle cleansing of the area once or twice a day with a liquid cleanser such as Cetaphil Lotion Cleanser, but don't clean the area in the shower, where a high-pressure shower-head might irritate the skin; and keep the area moist with a moisturizer, Vaseline, or antibiotic ointment.

It's extremely important that you don't pick at the skin or disturb any scabs or crusts that form in any way. Picking or disturbing the healing process may create scarring. Be sure to tell your doctor if any blisters or scabs have formed. These will usually heal just fine with proper treatment, but you may be asked to use a different type of dressing on those areas. Also, immediately report any pus, yellow crusts, redness with tenderness associated with it, or fever. Infections following cosmetic treatments are rare, but they do occasionally occur and need to be treated promptly.

Mild bruising or redness at treatment sites isn't uncommon, but let your doctor know if you think it's excessive. Any marks or discolorations that may result from your treatment will usually heal within a week. (The exception, of course, is full-face laser resurfacing, which takes much longer to completely heal.) Another exception is if you should develop brown spots at treatment sites. This is called *post-inflammatory hyperpigmentation* and can sometimes take months or even a year or more to resolve. Be sure to let your dermatologist know if that happens because you may be asked to use special treatment products.

Treatments in Series

"I'm very red from rosacea, and my doctor recommended approximately five treatments. Do I really need this many?"

Many laser and cosmetic treatments are now performed in a series of fairly gentle treatments for which there is no downtime. A photorejuvenation series for rosacea or sun damage, for instance, usually requires approximately five treatments. The interval between treatments tends to be a minimum of three or four weeks. Most dermatologists don't have a problem with the interval being extended longer than that, but be sure to discuss it with your particular doctor. (Just remember that the longer your intervals are, the slower your progress will be.)

Get the Most from Your Laser Treatments

You'll be investing a considerable amount of time and money to improve your skin, so here's how to maximize your treatments:

1. Give those consent forms and pretreatment instructions your full attention; that way, you won't do things such as take Advil the night before your treatment.

2. Get your questions answered *before* the treatment. Saving a lot of questions for the treatment shortens the time the nurse, physician's assistant, or doctor has for your treatment itself.

3. Follow the post-treatment instructions to the letter. If you just can't live without your run or yoga, call the nurse first and make sure you're not jeopardizing the success of your treatment.

Long-Term Expectations

"Will I require any maintenance treatments after I'm cleared up?"

Yes. Nothing is truly permanent. After all, you'll still be getting some sun even if you're careful, you're still aging, and . . . no one has perfect health habits. Expect to need some maintenance treatments after your initial treatment series—this is true of photorejuvenation, treatments for leg veins, hair removal, and almost everything else. Ask your doctor what to expect in this area.

Maintenance for photorejuvenation (for redness, rosacea, brown and age spots, or fine wrinkles) is normally done every six to twelve months depending on your particular problems or goals. After laser hair removal, you might expect anywhere from one to four maintenance treatments per year for a while. After removing many of the signs of sun damage with a gentle laser, microdermabrasion can be a relatively inexpensive way to maintain the gains.

Also, lifestyle makes a huge difference. If you're really scrupulous about using good-quality sunscreens every morning and avoiding the environmental stresses that aggravate your problem, you'll probably do very well over time and require little in the way of maintenance. If, on the other hand, you love to ski at high altitudes and sometimes forget to put your sunscreen on, you may need to have more frequent maintenance treatments.

DIFFERENT LASER SYSTEMS

"Each laser center I call seems to use a different system and thinks that theirs is the best. How do I know who's right?"

If you find this area confusing, you're not alone. In fact, many *doctors* who aren't involved with lasers find this area baffling. At present count, there are at least 20 different companies making laser systems, and many of them make anywhere from two to eight different types of laser systems.

Some of these companies (such as Lumenis, which is a merger of three fairly large laser companies), are large, well established, and have a long track record in the industry. Others are tiny companies with one laser system that's only been out for a year or so. Most of the laser machines on the market do what they're designed to; what matters much more is the training, judgment, experience, and ethics of the physician and physician-supervised personnel who are actually operating the laser.

Most larger laser centers in urban areas will have up-to-date equipment. You might want to ask about the equipment in smaller, more rural areas where there may be only one laser available. Laser equipment will usually last anywhere from three to eight years with excellent maintenance. For older machines, there are often upgrades that make them as current as any newer lasers on the market.

Marketing hype. There tends to be a lot of hoopla accompanying newer laser technology. Often this marketing hype isn't warranted, such as when the new equipment offers no particular advantage over what already exists.

Also, new lasers are often just a dressed-up version of an older laser. For example, alexandrite lasers are excellent for hair removal. Newer alexandrite lasers might have a new cooling tip or other bells and whistles, but the basic functionality of the machine remains the same.

Specific Lasers for Specific Problems

Lasers for redness and "broken" and enlarged blood vessels on the face. These lasers work by targeting hemoglobin, which is the red pigment in blood. The laser light is selectively absorbed by the blood in the tiny vessels in your skin. The blood heats up and damages the vessel, which then slowly dissolves and is reabsorbed by your own body. Thus, the redness and enlarged blood vessels slowly go away.

At present, there are at least 14 different companies making these vascular lasers. Some of the most commonly used are the MultiLight, the Quantum, the Vasculite, the Gentlelase, and the Versapulse.

Lasers for age spots and brown spots. These lasers work by targeting melanin, the pigment in our skin. Melanin is present in our skin in microscopic granules—a brown spot just has a higher density of those granules. Laser light is absorbed by and shatters the melanin granules into tiny microscopic particles. This debris is then carried away by your own immune system. (Tattoo removal works in a very similar way.)

Hair-reduction systems. These lasers also work by targeting melanin, which is the dark pigment in the hair shaft. The melanin in the hair absorbs the laser light, which then heats up the hair bulb that grows the hair at the base of the follicle. As the hair bulb and shaft of the hair heat up, the hair is injured and grows in more slowly (and often with a smaller, finer diameter). With repeated treatments and further injury, sometimes that follicle will even stop growing hair completely.

Hair-removal lasers work best if you have darker hair and lighter skin. The more contrast there is

between the hair color and the skin, the easier it is for the laser to find the hair follicle. If you have a darker skin type and a lot of melanin in the skin as well, the laser gets confused and it's easier for the laser to burn the skin.

It's very important if you have darker skin to go to a center where they have lots of experience treating darker skin types. (Yet even with experienced centers, there are sometimes complications, because everyone is an individual.) Also, if you've been out in the sun at all, it's extremely important to tell your doctor, as she may have to readjust the laser settings from the last visit.

Right now there are 17 different companies making laser hair-removal systems. Most centers are now using alexandrite lasers, diode lasers, or intense pulsed-light systems such as the EpiLight.

Laser treatment of sun damage and wrinkles. These treatments are often referred to as *photorejuvenation* or *non-ablative skin rejuvenation.* There are basically two different types of systems for this at present: One targets just the wrinkles and doesn't affect any blotchiness or discoloration you may have from sun damage; the other systems do all three. If your blotchiness is red or brown, see the first two sections above for how they work. As for fine wrinkles, all of these lasers work by heating up the cells deep in the skin (the *dermis*), called *fibroblasts,* which then produce more collagen.

Treatments are usually done in a series of about five sessions over a period of approximately five months. The skin then looks smoother with better texture and is more even in color. Be wary of any system that promises you wrinkle reduction in one or two treatments.

Lasers for leg veins. Until recently, most of the lasers available for this purpose didn't work very well, and most dermatologists continue to primarily use injections for the treatment of leg veins. The reason for this is that leg veins are larger and deeper than the veins on the face, and they have more pressure in them since they're lower down in the body. But several newer lasers with longer wavelengths (for example, the 1064 YAG) have proven to be effective in treating leg veins, and they also have an excellent safety profile in experienced hands.

Resurfacing lasers for deep wrinkles and acne scars. These lasers work by wearing away or removing the top layer of skin in a very carefully controlled manner. A new layer of "baby" skin then grows back. There hasn't been much change in these lasers in the past several years. CO_2 and erbium lasers are still most commonly used for this problem—they may have a few new features, but they're basically the same lasers that were being used several years ago. Both types of lasers offer excellent results in experienced hands.

Sometimes these lasers will be used together, with a CO_2 laser being used first, followed by one or two passes of an erbium laser. Erbium lasers help to speed healing time and diminish the redness that usually follows CO_2 laser resurfacing, and they're most appropriately used for certain types of acne scarring or moderate to severe wrinkles.

෧෧ ෧෧ ෧෧   ෧෧ ෧෧ ෧෧

PART II

—◇—

COLOR PROBLEMS

5

BROWN SPOTS
AND AGE SPOTS

Some of the most frequent questions I hear from patients relate to the spots they notice on their faces and hands: "What are these? Are they freckles? Why am I getting them? How can I get rid of them? Will they turn into huge liver spots like on my grandmother's hands?"

This chapter will provide you with the basics on these kinds of spots so that you can understand your own, and it will also describe the various treatments that help make these spots fade or disappear.

WHAT YOU NEED TO KNOW

- Sun damage
- Age spots
- Skin color and type
- Brown patches (melasma)
- Birthmarks
- Skin diseases

WHAT ARE THE POSSIBLE TREATMENTS?

- Bleaching creams
- Lasers
- Chemical peels
- Glycolic peels and micro-dermabrasion
- Liquid nitrogen
- Resurfacing laser peels

WHAT YOU NEED TO KNOW

Sun Damage

"My older sister keeps telling me that I look sun damaged. What does this mean?"

Compare the skin of a very young child with the skin on your face, and you'll be able to instantly understand what your sister's talking about. The skin of a child radiates a translucent glow, appears uniform in color, and is smooth in texture. By the time we're 30 to 40, many of us have a few age spots or brown spots, some blotchiness or redness, dry or even leathery texture, and some sagging or wrinkling. Most of that comes from sun damage, or *photoaging*.

And if you think your skin looks the way it does due to normal aging, check out the skin on your face versus the skin on your body that's been protected from the sun (for example, the skin on your breasts or on the inside of your thighs). Those protected areas are what your face would look like without sun damage. Age certainly etches lines of expression into the face and causes the skin to eventually lose some elasticity, but prolonged exposure to sunlight is what dramatically accelerates the aging process.

You've probably heard about UVA and UVB radiation, which are the two types of ultraviolet light from the sun that cause damage to our skin. Until fairly recently, doctors thought that most damage was caused only by UVB light. But now we know that UVA light also causes photoaging and contributes to skin cancer.

UVB is a shorter wavelength of light and is strongest between 11:00 A.M. and 3:00 P.M. It's sometimes called the "burning ray" because it's responsible for most sunburns— and sunburns, especially in childhood, have been linked to the deadliest type of skin cancer we know of—melanoma.

UVA radiation has longer wavelengths than UVB, which may cause fewer burns, but penetrate further into the skin, do more damage to the collagen and elastic fibers, and generate wrinkles and skin cancers. Tanning booths use UVA light— sure, they may not give you a sunburn, but they'll definitely expose you to sun damage and risk. UVA radiation also penetrates clouds and the windows of your car, office, and home. It's much more constant throughout the day and year than UVB, which peaks during the midday and in the summer.

The sun is even riskier at high elevations (Denver, for example) or when you're skiing, hiking, or mountain climbing. Sunlight causes more damage on the water, too— the light reflected off the water just adds to regular direct sunlight. If you're using a sunscreen that blocks UVB but not UVA, you won't be protected from a lot of the damage that the light is doing to your skin.

To prevent sun damage, including age spots and brown spots, you should use a sunscreen that blocks both UVA and UVB light. The SPF rating you see on sunscreens covers *only* UVB. Look for sunscreens that say "broad spectrum" and have zinc, Parsol 1789/avobenzone, or titanium. Of course, the sunscreens that block both UVA and UVB radiation can be a little more expensive, but if you really want to prevent the spots, wrinkles, and blotchiness that the sun causes, then you need to block them both.

Suntans and fashion. For Caucasian women, suntans have been fashionable for more than half a century now. But it was not always so. For hundreds of years before World War II, the most prized complexion was a fair one. Such words as *porcelain* and *alabaster* denoted beautiful skin in the United States and Northern Europe. Today, as American baby boomers have aged, and the wrinkling and drying effects of the sun have become more obvious, there's been a slow shift in our cultural conception of beauty back to a less-bronzed appearance.

Age Spots

"I'm only 37, so why am I already getting age spots?"

Allow me to clear up one misconception here: Age spots are a misnomer—they really should be called *sun spots*.

These spots usually occur first on our faces and on the backs of our hands. In Victorian times, ladies prevented the spots by wearing bonnets and gloves, which is perhaps a bit extreme for today's active lifestyles, but if we thoroughly protected ourselves from the sun, we wouldn't have any age spots. And, yes, it's

quite possible to develop them at a young age, even in your 30s. This is especially true if you have red or blonde hair and very fair skin.

The first goal is to prevent development of more of these spots by using lots of sunscreen containing zinc or avobenzone. Many women now wisely use sunscreen on their faces, chests, and necks every morning to help prevent sun damage. The hands, however, present a different challenge, because sunscreen often washes off when we wash our hands. A water-resistant, sweat-resistant, high-SPF sunscreen will help. If you've had precancerous lesions or skin cancer on your hands, you might even want to consider keeping sunscreen in the glove compartment of your car and in your purse so that you can reapply it frequently.

Another strategy is to use gloves as frequently as possible. In cool climates this makes sense; buy them in basic and fun colors and keep them everywhere. But if you live in a warm, sunny climate, sunscreen is probably your best option for prevention.

Golfers frequently get age spots on the hand that isn't gloved. If you engage in this sport, try playing with gloves on both hands to keep the skin color even, or apply waterproof sunscreen to your ungloved hand.

Skin Color and Type

"I'm African-American and have noticed that my skin is getting blotchier as time goes on. What's causing this? Do I need to wear sunscreen?"

The most common causes of blotchiness in all skin types are sun damage; acne or other skin diseases; and melasma, which is caused by pregnancy, oral contraceptives, or hormone replacement therapy.

Darker skin types will often notice temporary marks after injury or inflammation of the skin. For example, a cut may initially heal with a dark stripe that will usually resolve in time. By the same token, acne that causes inflammation in the skin will often leave a dark mark that may take months to resolve.

If you have acne or other skin diseases, it's very important to treat the condition as quickly as possible to avoid leaving these marks (called *post-inflammatory hyperpigmentation*). Also, if you're taking oral contraceptives, you may want to ask your dermatologist whether your pills could be aggravating this problem. Oral contraceptives can be helpful for acne, but they can also cause a type of brown discoloration called *melasma*. (Other birth-control methods don't tend to affect the skin.)

Sun damage can occur in African-American skin just as it does in other skin types. Skin pigment, or melanin, is a natural sunscreen, and is present in greater amounts the darker your skin is. But melanin doesn't protect you completely, and, if you've spent a lot of time in the sun and are getting blotchy, the sun may indeed be the culprit.

In order to rid your skin of blotchiness, try these steps:

1. Get any skin diseases such as acne treated by your dermatologist.

2. Wear an SPF 15 or higher sunscreen with zinc or avobenzone/Parsol 1789 in it every morning.

3. Talk to your doctor about stopping or changing your oral contraceptives, or discuss another birth-control method.

4. Try nonprescription "bleaching" creams, which are 2-percent hydroquinone, for one or two months. If that's not helping, ask your dermatologist for a prescription-strength bleaching cream.

Brown Patches (Melasma)

"I had brown spots develop on my skin during my first pregnancy, but they went away after I delivered. While pregnant with my second child, the same thing happened—but this time, they don't seem to be going away. Why is this happening?"

Pregnancy is a common cause of brown spots or blotches, which doctors call *melasma,* on all skin types. In fact, melasma can appear anytime a woman's hormones change—whether due to pregnancy, the use of oral contraceptives, or hormone replacement therapy after menopause. All of these situations can stimulate a hormone that tells the skin to make more pigment, which, in combination with light, can produce too much pigment. The result is often brown blotchy patches, usually across the cheeks or on the forehead—but the neck, chest, or back can develop them as well.

Once melasma has gotten started (during a pregnancy, for example), it may become very difficult to treat. If you do develop melasma while pregnant, chances are it will resolve itself after you deliver, but it may recur with subsequent pregnancies, particularly if you're expecting during the summer. And in a small percentage of women, melasma just gets worse over time and with exposure to sunlight.

The first strategy with melasma is to try to prevent it in the first place. If you're pregnant, particularly in the summer, be sure to apply a high-SPF sunscreen with zinc or avobenzone every single morning and reapply it frequently. (You should also wear a hat.)

If the melasma is being caused by your oral contraceptive and it's bothering you, then you should probably find another method of birth control. Melasma resulting from oral contraceptives usually becomes worse over time and increasingly difficult to treat.

Hormone-replacement therapy (HRT) is a bit trickier, as many women may not be able to simply stop taking the hormone due to health reasons. It may help to take the estrogen in the evening instead of the morning so that peak levels occur during the night and not when you might be out in the light. You can also try changing from a pill to a skin patch, as your body may absorb the estrogen through the patch without the peaks and valleys that sometimes occur when taking oral medication. This may not work for all women, but it's worth a try if you really need to keep taking estrogen. Changing to a lower dose may also help.

Again, use sunscreen, stay out of the midday sun, and keep your hat on. Ask your dermatologist about prescription "bleaching" creams, or consider changing your contraception or your hormone replacement therapy. All of these simple measures will help to limit the blotchiness of melasma.

"I have melasma, and my doctor told me to use sunscreen every day. The melasma keeps getting worse even when I'm doing that. Why?"

Remember that even the best sunscreen doesn't block all ultraviolet light—so, despite your best efforts, it's that small amount getting through your sunscreen that's activating your melasma.

The only way to block the light completely is to wear protective clothing or use the zinc compound that lifeguards and mountain climbers often use on their noses and cheeks. But few people want to go to that extreme. Here are less-extreme (and still effective) measures you can take:

1. Wash your face, let it dry for a few minutes, and then put on a sunscreen containing avobenzone (such as Cetaphil Daily Facial Moisturizer).

2. Let that dry, and then apply a high-quality sunscreen containing zinc over that. Sometimes layering avobenzone with zinc provides a little bit of extra protection.

3. Be sure that you're using enough sunscreen. The most common mistake that people make in this area is they don't apply it thickly enough. To cover your entire face well, you should be using about two teaspoons.

4. If you're going to sweat or partic-ipate in water sports, then the sunscreen you're using should be waterproof and sweatproof—you don't want to wash it off the minute you go swimming.

5. You can apply your foundation on top if you wish, but make sure that it's SPF 15—and be aware that most people don't apply foundation thick enough for it to be protective on its own.

Keep in mind that wide-brimmed hats make a big difference, since they screen almost all the direct light coming from above, and the only light hitting your face is what's reflected off the ground, water, or objects around you. Also, if you're not self-conscious, you could get the completely opaque climbers' sunscreen and use that on your melasma spots.

Why Melasma Is So Tough to Treat

Melasma is the name for those blotchy, brown patches that show up most commonly in pregnancy. The hormones of pregnancy stimulate the growth of cells that make brown pigment (melanocytes). And natural light stimulates the production of even more brown pigment (melanin). Estrogens in oral contraceptives and hormone replacement therapy can also do this. So you have two problems: too many cells making brown pigment, and light con-stantly stimulating them. Here's what to do:

1. Use the best quality sunscreen possible every morning (think zinc and SPF 30 or higher).
2. Wear a wide-brimmed hat.
3. Try bleaching creams from your dermatologist (the strong ones require a prescription).
4. Get a series of microdermabrasion or light peels, which, if done correct-ly, can help reduce the discoloration.
5. If you can, change your contraception method or decrease your estro-gen dose.

Birthmarks

"I have a large brown birthmark on my upper back. Can this be removed?"

Some brown birthmarks are at higher risk for developing skin can-cers, so have your dermatologist

check it. Assuming that it's been checked and is fine, many birth-marks smaller than a half-dollar can be surgically removed, and red birthmarks can now be removed or improved with laser treatment. (Check with your dermatologist to see if you have a type of birthmark that's safe to treat with a laser.)

Before you have your birthmark removed, ask yourself two questions: (1) Is the scar better than the birthmark itself? and (2) is the birthmark part of what makes you distinctive? A birthmark can be a mark of individuality, a signature on your skin—do you really want to get rid of it?

Following is a list of the most common types of birthmarks, along with information on whether they can be removed or not.

— Most brown spots that people consider birthmarks are, in fact, moles. One that grows a lot of hair is called a *Beckers nevus*. If such a mole is small and in a spot where a scar won't show, it may be reasonable to have it surgically removed. Larger ones may be treated with a laser to remove the hair, but the mole itself should usually be left alone. Consult your dermatologist for her recommendation.

— Flat, light, coffee-colored birthmarks are called *café-au-lait spots*, after the milky coffee served in France. These can occur either singly or in multiples almost anywhere on the body, and can be just about any size. Small spots are fine, but if you have several large ones, you should ask your doctor about them, since having a lot of these spots can occasionally be an indicator of certain genetic diseases. In addition, sunlight tends to darken them over time.

— There's also a type of mole that looks like a lot of little polka dots right next to each other. These can be quite large and found anywhere on the body. Generally, they don't cause any problems, even though they might be cosmetically annoying. They can be surgically removed if they're small.

— Larger moles are at an increased risk for developing *melanoma* (the skin cancer that can become very serious). These should be carefully monitored by a dermatologist, who may very well surgically remove them so that they won't cause problems later.

— A type of mole often found on the face in Asian populations is called the *Nevus of Ota*. This type of birthmark can sometimes be successfully removed with lasers.

— Red or purplish birthmarks (called *port-wine stains*) can be improved or removed with lasers now. Ask your dermatologist about this.

You should also watch your birthmark to see if it changes, and have your primary-care doctor or your dermatologist check it, too. It's also not a bad idea to take a photograph of the birthmark yearly and keep it on file. Then if there's any question in your mind that it may have changed, you can compare it to the photo. If you have any questions, see your dermatologist, and take the photographs with you.

Protect birthmarks from the sun by applying a high-SPF sunscreen containing zinc every day.

"Can lasers remove birthmarks?"

Lasers *can* technically remove

some brown birthmarks, but the question is whether they can do so safely. The concern is that the laser might in some way cause the melanocytes (the cells that make skin pigment) in the birthmark to transform and increase the risk of cancer years later. So far, there's been no evidence of this, but we don't have much long-term data on the subject. Until there are studies done that show safety over a long period, I don't recommend lasers for removing most brown birthmarks, but they do work well on brown spots caused by sun damage.

Skin Diseases

"I have both eczema and acne. Every time I get a pimple or an outbreak of eczema, it leaves a brown spot after it heals, which can sometimes last for months. Is there anything I can do about this?"

Acne, eczema, and even cuts all create wounds in the skin. And when white blood cells rush to a wound to help it heal, they also stimulate pigment formation . . . sometimes too much. The pigment clumps together, resulting in the brown spots you describe. Imagine that your body is a quarterback throwing not one, but eight or ten balls all at once to the receiver. The receiver can't catch all ten balls, so they drop nearby and just sit there in a brown clump. The medical term for this process is *post-inflammatory hyperpigmentation.*

These brown spots tend to occur primarily in people with darker skin or dark hair and brown eyes. The first thing to do is get the acne and eczema under control by seeing a dermatologist. Sunscreen will also help prevent and limit these spots—use a high-SPF sunscreen containing zinc for your best success.

The good news is that these types of brown spots will usually resolve on their own. They can also be treated and prevented in many instances with various creams. Some that are known to be helpful include hydroquinone, tretinoin, azelaic acid, kojic acid, topical steroids, and possibly certain creams containing plant extracts such as arbutin and thymol. Microdermabrasion also helps. Sometimes lasers can be used if protective measures, skin-lightening creams, light peels, and microdermabrasion are unsuccessful.

You'll want to work closely with a dermatologist if you have this problem, since most of the treatments I've mentioned require a doctor's care or a prescription.

What Are the Possible Treatments?

Bleaching Creams

"My doctor prescribed a bleaching cream to help with the brown spots I have. Will this really bleach my skin?"

No. These creams don't really bleach anything; instead, they block the production of excess pigment in the skin. So when your skin cells regenerate, lighter normal pigment will gradually replace the brown pigment.

Here's how it works. The pigment-making cells in your skin are like little factories that churn out microscopic brown granules. The amount and shade of brown depends on your skin type, which you inherited from your family. Bleaching creams partially shut down the factory, so less brown pigment granules are made. However, as soon as you stop using the cream, especially if you aren't careful with sunscreen, light stimulates the factory, and pigment production may gear up again, causing your problem to recur.

Bleaching creams do a good job of lightening brown discoloration. The one most commonly prescribed is hydroquinone in a 4-percent concentration. (Two-percent creams are available without a prescription.) Hydroquinone is the generic name, and it has several trade names as well. Some of the most commonly used prescription hydroquinones are Lustra, Lustra-AF, Alustra, Claripel, or Tri-Luma.

Lustra cream is a 4-percent hydroquinone in a base that's pleasant to use and smells good (many hydroquinone creams smell awful). Lustra-AF and Alustra have glycolic acid and retinol added to them respectively to speed up the lightening process. But if the standard hydroquinone creams aren't working for you, your dermatologist may recommend a stronger, specially compounded mixture, such as 6-percent hydroquinone.

Other creams that are used as sole lightening agents or in combination are tretinoin, azelaic acid, and alpha-hydroxy acid. These creams work by speeding up cell turnover. (Kojic acid and plant extracts such as arbutin and thymol inhibit pigment production, at least in laboratory tests.)

Lasers

"My dermatologist suggested using a laser to remove the age spots on my face. I understand that there are a lot of different types of lasers now for this. Could you explain the differences to me?"

In the hands of the right practitioner, lasers are safe and effective ways to remove age spots and brown spots, and they require very little patient downtime.

But the number of lasers and laser practitioners has greatly increased in the last ten years, and lasers are powerful machines. The best way to ensure that you get the safest and most effective treatment is to be treated in a dermatologist's office by a physician or nurse who is an expert in laser therapy.

"How do lasers work?"

Lasers send a concentrated beam of light, which travels from the laser machine through a cord into a handset held by the practitioner, who passes the handset over the skin to be treated. The treatment is done in a doctor's office.

Certain lasers, most suitable for age spots and brown spots, use their beams of light to destroy the pigment that gives the spots their brown color. The more powerful resurfacing lasers actually burn off a thin layer of skin. When the skin heals, it repairs itself with new, undamaged skin.

If you have moderate to severe sun damage and deeper wrinkles along with your age spots, the more powerful resurfacing laser peel may be your best choice. But if your main targets are age spots and brown spots, then choose a gentler laser that doesn't break the skin and heals much faster. Two good options are the MultiLight, which uses intense pulsed light (a close cousin to a laser), or the Nd:YAG. Compared to resurfacing lasers, these treatments are usually less expensive, have less risk of complications, and require less downtime. Let's look at those first and then discuss the more powerful resurfacing lasers.

Photorejuvenation is done with an intense pulsed light device (also known as IPL, MultiLight, or PhotoDerm). These "laser cousins" use light that's passed through a filter in the handpiece of the IPL. The practitioner passes the handset over the skin being treated, and the light from the laser hits the brown spots and damages the melanin, or brown pigment, creating a light crust. The age or sun spots look slightly darker for about a week and then begin to lighten and sometimes peel. The laser treatment is usually repeated three to five times depending on the number of the age spots and how dark they are. It's possible to use makeup right after the treatment, but some physicians prefer that patients wait a number of days before doing so.

These aren't considered "true" lasers by the FDA, but they do in fact function like lasers. Everyone in the room, whether patient or medical personnel, should always wear laser goggles or special contact lenses at the time of this treatment.

Nd:YAG laser. The Nd:YAG laser has been used for many years in the treatment of brown spots and age spots and also does an excellent job. Be sure to distinguish between Nd:YAG lasers used for age spots and Erbium:YAG lasers used for resurfacing. As with the IPL lasers above, age spots will often crust slightly for a week to two weeks and then peel off, a series is more effective than just one treatment, and per-treatment costs are usually similar.

Both IPL and Nd:YAG laser treatments are done in the dermatologist's office, usually without intravenous anesthetic. Often these treatments are so gentle that no anesthetic is needed at all; sometimes topical anesthetic cream (such as ELA-Max) may be used, or possibly a small injection of a local anesthetic.

The cost for laser treatment of age spots and brown spots varies according to your doctor, the region you live in, and the number and degree of darkness of the spots being treated. But the range for the treatment of face or hands is approximately $300 to $700 per session, with three to five treatments usually being necessary to achieve desired results.

Chemical Peels

"I live in a small town in the Midwest, and there are no laser specialists nearby. My dermatologist suggested a trichloroacetic acid peel and said that it would be similar to a light laser peel. Do you

think this is a good idea?"

Dermatologists have been using trichloroacetic acid (TCA), a cousin to vinegar, to do chemical peeling for at least 15 years. Some dermatologists, in fact, still prefer TCA to laser peels. A TCA peel is excellent and safe in the hands of an experienced professional, and is a good option, especially in areas where laser peels might not be available. The cost generally ranges from $400 to $2,000 depending on how deep the peel is, your doctor, and where you live.

One of the main advantages of a TCA peel is that it can easily be done in your dermatologist's office. It doesn't require an anesthesiologist to be present or any intravenous anesthesia. Often physicians give patients a little bit of Valium prior to the procedure. For any discomfort during or after the peel, acetaminophen, Vioxx, or other anti-inflammatories work well, but there are many other options. Some physicians allow their patients to apply lidocane (a light topical anesthetic) prior to the procedure, and most will also have a nurse hold a fan close to the patient's face during a short period in the procedure when there's a sensation of heat.

The other advantage of a TCA peel is that its concentration can be adjusted to achieve lighter or deeper peels depending on your skin type and goals. For example, your physician might use a lower strength around the eyes and the jawline and a higher strength around the mouth or any areas with more sun damage.

There's also a pre-peel solution called *Jessner's solution,* which can be applied before the procedure and allows the TCA to penetrate better, thus giving a slightly deeper and more even peel. Your physician will decide whether that's a good idea for you. (Sometimes Jessner's solution is used alone as a light peeling agent.)

The disadvantage of the TCA peel is that everyone's skin is different. Even areas on the same face are different—occasionally, one area will take up the peel solution much more strongly than other areas, which causes a small erosion or blister. These generally heal fine without any scarring. In fact, problems with scarring are very rare, but occasionally there are red areas that may take several months to resolve.

The other disadvantage is that a TCA peel can be mildly to moderately uncomfortable since no intravenous anesthesia is used. However, with good pre-op medications, discomfort is usually minimal and lasts only five to ten minutes.

Get the Best Results from Your TCA Peel

Since you're investing precious time and money in your skin, you'll want to get the very best results and the fastest healing time possible. Here are some hints to speed your healing.

1. If you're a smoker, stop or cut way back (at least temporarily), because smoking robs the skin of oxygen, and cells won't regenerate as quickly.

2. Really beef up your nutrition by getting at least 50 grams of protein a day during the month prior to your peel. (You may feel so good that you'll keep it up!)

3. Be sure that your multivitamin has zinc in it, which is known to promote wound healing.

4. Use Renova for one to two months before the peel, for it's been shown to speed up healing by increasing cell regeneration and smoothing the outer cell layers so the peel takes more evenly. Most dermatologists will have you stop the Renova a week before the TCA peel, so be sure to ask your doctor for instructions.

5. If you have a history of cold sores (herpes simplex), be sure to let your dermatologist know. You'll be given medication to take before and during the healing phase to prevent an outbreak.

Glycolic Peels and Microdermabrasion

"I'm in my 30s and have red hair. I already have a number of age spots on my face, which my dermatologist suggested should be treated with microdermabrasion or glycolic peels. Should I spend my money on a deeper chemical peel, or will the lighter peels do a good job for me?"

This is a little difficult to answer without seeing you. But generally, if you have light to moderate sun damage, have some freckling or light age spots, and are in your 30s, light peels or microdermabrasion are an excellent way to go.

Glycolic peels and microdermabrasion, despite their somewhat scary names, are light peels. A glycolic peel is a very mild chemical peel that uses an acid derived from sugarcane. Microdermabrasion smooths the skin by blowing tiny crystals against it to even its surface. Sometimes both processes can be combined to get a slightly deeper peel.

Both glycolic peels and microdermabrasion are usually done in a series of five to ten treatments depending on how many brown spots and how much sun damage you have. The cost is significantly less than with deeper peels (generally between $75 and $200 per peel depending on where you live), and the skin is usually slightly pink bordering on light red for one to four days depending on what was used.

These light peels, especially when used in conjunction with bleaching creams, often yield excellent results in younger women or men. Please find a dermatologist who has a closely supervised and experienced nurse or aesthetician to do these peels, for serious complications, while rare, can occur.

Light peels and microdermabrasion can also be excellent maintenance tools after laser treatments or chemical peels. A microdermabrasion treatment every few months may help maintain the improvement in skin texture, color, and wrinkling. But be sure to wait until your dermatologist gives you permission to begin these treatments if you've had recent laser or chemical peels.

Liquid Nitrogen

"My doctor suggested liquid nitrogen to get rid of brown spots on my hands. What do you think?"

For many years, liquid nitrogen was the main treatment available for treating age spots. The main drawback to this treatment is its tendency to leave white areas or uneven blotchy areas after the spot is treated. For this reason, most dermatologists who do a lot of cosmetic dermatology don't tend to use liquid nitrogen as much now. Other treatments provide a better, more even result in the long run.

Resurfacing Laser Peels

"I have a lot of age spots and wrinkles, and my dermatologist recommended a resurfacing laser peel for me. Is this a good idea?"

If your only goal is removing age spots, then the gentler lasers mentioned above will generally be a better option for you than a resurfacing (CO_2) peel. They're less expensive, less risky, and there's less downtime associated with them.

However, if your spots are associated with moderate to severe sun damage and deeper wrinkles, then a resurfacing laser may be a great option—you can then take care of everything at the same time.

One advantage of CO_2 peels is that they allow the physician to make very accurate adjustments in the depth of the treatment. For example, a 42-year-old woman with only moderate sun damage may require just a light resurfacing, with a little more depth on upper-lip wrinkles; but a 52-year-old woman with old acne scarring, significant wrinkling, and sun damage may require a deeper laser treatment all over. A resurfacing laser peel can be customized to a woman's individual skin and goals.

CO_2 peels do have some significant downsides. First, they tend to be expensive (usually in the $4,000 to $8,000 range depending on where you live and your dermatologist). Second, they require significant time away from work and your usual activities (usually two to three weeks depending on the depth of the peel). For deeper peels, most dermatologists use an anesthesiologist to administer an intravenous sedative so that the procedure itself isn't uncomfortable. Expect mild to moderate discomfort in the first days of healing after the procedure, which can be managed with prescription pain medication. Swelling and oozing last approximately three to five days. An experienced dermatologic laser surgeon will manage your postoperative period closely to minimize discomfort and complications. And most patients will be red for one to six months afterwards, with some pinkness occasionally lingering after that.

Resurfacing laser peels are a significant surgery, and I ask patients to think of them as nonsurgical face-lifts and to act accordingly.

Summary of Brown Spots and Age Spots: What to Do

Let's assume that you have a few age spots or brown spots on your face and several on each hand. Your dermatologist has confirmed that they're from sun damage and aren't skin cancer or some other serious skin problem. You want to get rid of these spots, but you don't have the deep wrinkles that would call for a deep laser peel or resurfacing. Here's what you may want to consider:

- Always use a good **sunscreen** that blocks UVA and UVB. Even if you get rid of the brown spots, continued sun exposure will likely bring them right back.

- Try a **bleaching cream** prescribed by your doctor—the cost is minimal and the results can be excellent. (Remember to protect the treated area from the sun.)

- If the bleaching creams don't work to your satisfaction, try a **light chemical peel** or **microdermabrasion**. A series of three to five treatments may remove the spots at a cost per treatment of $75 to $200 depending on where you live and your doctor.

- Try the gentle **lasers,** such as the intense pulsed light (IPL) or the Nd:YAG. These can yield excellent results in three to five treatments with no downtime for you. But be prepared to pay $300 to $700 per treatment depending on where you live and your doctor.

- **Liquid nitrogen** is an option, but it's used less now because it sometimes leaves unsightly white areas after it heals.

Be sure to talk to your dermatologist about any suspicious spots, and seek out an experienced laser dermatologist.

෨ ෨ ෨   ෨ ෨ ෨

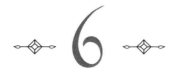

PROBLEMS
WITH RED SKIN

Problems with red skin have bedeviled women for generations. For some, redness runs in the family, particularly those with Celtic genes; for others, redness comes from hormonal changes or plain old sun damage. There's no blanket solution to this problem, but let's look at the different causes and see what can be done to reduce redness or get rid of it completely.

WHAT ARE THE POSSIBLE CAUSES?

- Rosacea
- Repeated flushing and blushing
- Sun damage
- Alcohol
- Exercise
- Coffee
- Hormones
- Allergies
- Your family history

WHAT ARE THE POSSIBLE TREATMENTS?

- Lifestyle changes
- Lasers
- Nonprescription creams
- Propranolol and clonidine

POSSIBLE CAUSES

"What causes redness?"

The red you see on your face is predominantly created by tiny blood vessels in the skin dilating. All of us, of course, have vessels that supply blood to our skin—but in many people, those blood vessels are more numerous, bigger, and in some cases, closer to the surface than in others. (These extra blood vessels aren't needed for the health of your skin.) Over time, with repeated flushing and sun damage—which also causes dilation of the superficial blood vessels—those blood vessels can get quite large and become permanently dilated.

Generally, people with light skin and a tendency to freckle are more likely to get red as time goes on. And adults who are red often have a history of flushing and blushing easily as children. In addition, if you have a problem with redness as an adult, it's likely that you also turn bright red on hot days or when you exercise. The good news is that most of the time, redness isn't related to any serious underlying medical condition. Even *rosacea* (a type of adult acne characterized by redness that slowly worsens each year and gradually becomes permanent) can be diagnosed and treated very readily.

Rosacea

"I've flushed my whole life, and now I have red bumps on my face that look like acne. What is this?"

It's very likely to be rosacea, which can look red and bumpy like acne, or can appear as a red patch that's sometimes slightly puffy.

Rosacea is often called "adult-onset acne" because it often begins between the ages of 30 and 50. But rosacea is treated differently from acne. Unlike teenage acne, which appears first in the "T-zone" of the forehead, nose, and chin, rosacea is most common on the nose and upper cheeks. (It can also involve the eyes and chin.)

The good news is that rosacea can often be treated with creams rather than oral medicines. Most cases can be cleared up or controlled within several months.

"I've heard of triggers for rosacea. Can I lessen my redness without medical treatment?"

Rosacea can be triggered by a number of factors, and many patients can reduce their redness by doing some detective work to figure out their own personal triggers. The most common ones are alcohol and heat; but exercise, coffee, and some foods can also trigger redness.

Of course it's important to enjoy your life, but do you really need those five cups of coffee a day? Maybe one in the morning and one right after lunch would be plenty. No one should give up their exercise program because of redness, but perhaps doing yoga in a 110-degree room is not the best choice of exercise for you. Think creatively about the things that might be aggravating your rosacea, and then try to cut down or eliminate some of them. Every little bit that you can do will help over the long term.

Remember that rosacea is a disease that starts in midlife and often continues for 10, 20, or sometimes even 30 years, so the little things that you do every day really do make a difference over many years in the progression and treatment of this problem.

Repeated Flushing and Blushing

"I've been embarrassed by blushing ever since I was a child. Is this something I have to live with?"

If you were teased as a child because you flushed and blushed when you were embarrassed or nervous, then you're well aware of how unpleasant and difficult this problem can be. Even as adults, many people who flush or blush will avoid public speaking, or situations where their blushing becomes noticeable.

Interestingly, most people who suffer from flushing and blushing, as well as rosacea, have some Celtic genes in them. The Celts originated in England, Scotland, Ireland, and Wales, although their genetic influence is also apparent in other areas of Europe. In America, many people who aren't predominantly of Celtic origin still have the genes in their family history and may have inherited that tendency toward redness.

There's nothing that will eliminate flushing and blushing com-

pletely, but there are a number of options that can improve the condition.

Treatment. The first step in treating flushing and blushing is to search for and remove any dietary or environmental agents that may be aggravating the problem. Spicy foods, alcohol, coffee, tea, sunlight, sulfite preservatives in fresh fruits and vegetables, and monosodium glutamate should be avoided if you flush or blush after exposure to them.

Sometimes a medication called *propranalol* (in the class of medications called *beta-blockers*) might be prescribed at 10 to 20 milligrams three times a day before meals—or sometimes just before events (such as speeches) that cause flushing. Don't use this treatment if you have asthma or certain heart problems.

Another medication, clonidine, may be used, usually at 25 to 75 milligrams twice a day. This medication shouldn't be discontinued suddenly—it must be tapered under a doctor's supervision. It inhibits the blood vessels' ability to dilate.

Several other medications may be helpful, including antihistamines or propantheline bromide. Ask your dermatologist or primary-care doctor for an explanations of these agents.

Sun Damage

"I have redness on my neck and chest that seems to get worse in the sun. Could the sun be the culprit?"

Yes. Sunlight (ultraviolet radiation) causes the tiny blood vessels on the surface of the skin to dilate. You may see this effect as a red or reddish-brown discoloration or a lot of little broken blood vessels and red spots interspersed with brown areas on the face, neck, or chest area.

Hormones, in conjunction with the sun, can also slightly aggravate redness and blotchiness. Antibiotics such as tetracycline, doxycycline, and minocycline; and drugs for high blood pressure, particularly hydrochlorothiazide, can also make sun-exposed areas of your skin more sensitive to the sun. The medical term for this is *photosensitivity*.

The skin on the neck and chest is thin, so treating damaged skin in those areas can be difficult. You should be especially careful to avoid exposing those areas to lots of sun—keep them covered with a high-quality sunscreen containing zinc, or stay covered up.

Myths about Redness

1. **People with red noses are drinkers.**
   False. Many people with red noses or faces, particularly those of Irish, Scottish, or English descent, have rosacea or a genetic tendency toward redness. Alcohol can be a trigger for redness, but redness itself often has nothing to do with how much someone drinks.

2. **People who are red shouldn't exercise.**
   False. We all need exercise to stay healthy. The redness that occurs as a result of exercise isn't harmful, just annoying.

3. **People who are red have other health issues.**
   False. The vast majority of the time, being red isn't associated with any other more serious medical problem.

Alcohol

"Even when I have just one or two drinks, I turn bright red. Do I have to stop drinking?"

Even if you don't have rosacea, alcohol may not be your friend if you have a tendency toward redness. Alcohol dilates the blood vessels of the body, including the ones in the skin—so if you're already red or have that tendency, the flushing can be very noticeable. You could stop drinking completely, but if you really enjoy the occasional glass of wine, try doing the following things:

1. **Do some sleuthing on your alcohol use.** First, watch what happens when you drink. If you limit yourself to just one or two drinks per evening, do you still get red? If so, try eating some food with the alcohol to slow down the absorption.

Does it happen with all different types of alcohol or just some? Cheaper red wines and sulfites could be the culprits, so try drinking a higher quality red wine, white wine, or sulfite-free wine. You can also experiment with different spirits—some people can substitute vodka for gin, for example, and reduce their redness.

2. **Decrease your alcohol use.** One alcoholic drink a day, particularly with a meal, may have beneficial effects on fat levels. But there can be problems with drinking much more than that, especially for women, who are more susceptible to liver damage than men. Alcohol increases circulating estrogens in the blood, which may increase a women's risk of breast cancer; it also contributes to thinning of the bones (osteoporosis). And, as we all know, alcohol and pregnancy do not mix.

If the above measures fail, you may have to make a choice between alcohol and the redness in your skin.

Exercise

"I turn purple or bright red with exercise. Is this normal?"

Yes. It just means that the blood vessels close to the surface of your skin readily and visibly dilate when your heart rate and blood pressure go up. You may find that you exhibit the same flush with sexual activity, which is completely normal.

Exercise is vitally important for every organ in the body, including the skin. It improves the circulation and gives skin a healthy glow. Since it's important for you to keep exercising, try working out in cooler environments, and make sure that you cool down adequately afterwards. If you're exercising indoors, wear the lightest clothing that you feel comfortable in. If you live in a warmer climate, try exercising in the morning or evening to avoid the heat of midday. Wear layers so that you can shed them quickly to stay as cool as possible as you exercise.

Coffee

"I drink six cups of coffee a day. Do you think this could be aggravating my redness?"

Coffee, caffeinated teas, and even hot liquids can aggravate redness and rosacea in some people. There are so many health reasons now to cut down or eliminate coffee altogether that I think it's really worth considering. Here is the current evidence:

- One study in humans found that as little as one and a half to two cups of coffee a day could double the risk of miscarriage.

- Coffee has a diuretic effect and draws both fluid and calcium from the body. This is particularly important for women, many of whom are already calcium deficient and prone to osteoporosis.

- Caffeine may interfere with the absorption of iron, and many women are iron deficient.

- Caffeine, especially when taken late in the day, may interfere with adequate sleep.

• Tea, coffee (especially when used with cream and sugar), and colas are filling without being nutritious and may add unnecessary calories.

Hormones

"I seem much redder now that I'm pregnant. Will this go away after I deliver?"

Those pregnancy hormones induce a lot of physical changes, including changes in your skin. Blood vessels become more noticeable all over the body, especially in the face, breasts, and legs. You may even notice that the palms of your hands and the soles of your feet are redder. Fortunately, almost all of this will return to normal within several months of delivery. Only a small percentage of women stay red or go on to develop rosacea after pregnancy.

If you find yourself redder now during your pregnancy, you may want to avoid overheating. You may have scaled back your exercise program somewhat already depending on the month of your pregnancy, but in general, walking outdoors (if it's not too warm) doesn't aggravate the redness and is a wonderful way to keep your exercise program going while you're pregnant. Swimming in cool water is also a good way to get exercise without heating up too much. Again, the redness isn't permanent, and exercise is very important—so don't change good habits in order to avoid redness while you're pregnant.

"My doctor and I recently decided that hormone replacement would be the best option for me now that

I've gone through menopause. Since I've been on it, I've noticed that I'm redder. Is it my imagination?"

No, it's not your imagination. In a few women, higher doses of estrogens in particular can sometimes aggravate redness and blotchiness. If you notice an increase in redness in the sun, try taking your estrogen before you go to bed rather than in the morning to see if that makes a difference. In most women, the progesterone part of hormone replacement will aggravate acne but not melasma (brown discoloration) or redness.

Allergies

"I've noticed that my allergies are getting worse as I get older, and that I'm also getting redder. Could these be related?"

Allergies can definitely contribute to redness and dilated blood vessels. Many allergy sufferers are particularly red right around the base of the nose where they've been blowing or wiping their noses for many years. The constant mechanical irritations increase redness and blood vessels. If you suffer from allergies, you can limit the damage from wiping constantly by making sure the area is well lubricated with Vaseline or a cream such as Cetaphil or Eucerin, which acts as a lubricant and protects the skin from the wetting and drying effect.

There are also a number of skin allergies that can cause redness. Allergies to creams, soaps, and lotions, as well as to detergents and fabric softeners on pillowcases can cause redness and allergic reactions on the face. Allergies can also provoke eczema, which causes dry, often itchy, red, rough patches of skin—whereas redness associated with the other problems mentioned in this chapter isn't itchy or particularly uncomfortable.

Your Family History

"I'm 20 years old, and I've noticed that most adults in my family tend to be red and have rosacea. Does this mean that I'll probably get it, too?"

Yes, it probably does. Unfortunately, those genetic influences are quite strong, particularly if you have relatives on both sides of your family with redness and rosacea. If you have only one parent who has it, you may be lucky enough to get the genes from the side that isn't red. If there's a strong family history of rosacea and you're beginning to get red even in your 20s, you may want to see your doctor to discuss starting metronidazole cream, which is a common prescription remedy for rosacea.

POSSIBLE TREATMENTS

Lifestyle Changes

"Will lifestyle changes help me with my redness?"

Certain lifestyle changes may indeed help your redness, flushing and blushing, and rosacea. Not all changes will work for everyone, so experiment by making one change at a time. You'll want to try the change for at least several weeks before you decide if it's helping or not. Redness will often wax and wane over a period of weeks or months. If you try something for only a couple of days, you really can't be sure if it has made a difference or not. Following are some of the changes you might want to try:

- Avoid alcohol completely or try different types (for instance, white wine instead of red) to see if that makes a difference.

- If you have rosacea or aren't sure, see your dermatologist for diagnosis and treatment.

- If you live in a warm climate, exercise only in spaces that are 70 degrees or less—indoors or out.

- Try to steer clear of spicy foods.

- Avoid coffee and caffeinated teas.

- Drink warm (not hot) liquids.

- If you have allergies, make sure that they're treated and under control.

- If the sun seems to activate the redness, stay out of it or try using zinc-based sunscreens.

- If you think you might be perimenopausal or menopausal, check with your doctor to see if estrogen replacement is advisable for other reasons as well.

- If you're pregnant, avoid getting overheated or overly fatigued (a good idea anyway).

- If you're on hormone-replacement therapy already, try taking your estrogen at night instead of in the morning.

Treating Rosacea

"I was recently diagnosed with rosacea. If I use my medications, will my redness disappear?"

Not necessarily. If your rosacea is mild, or if you've only had it a short time, you may not be very red yet. In that case, your medications may be enough to control it.

But if you've had your rosacea a long time and are very red, even using all your medications faithfully probably won't resolve it. The medications will reduce the acne-like breakouts and over time help control the red and keep it from progressing, but they probably won't get rid of the redness you had *before* treatment. For that redness, gentle laser treatments are the best option for returning your face to its normal color.

Lasers

"I've gradually become redder and redder over the years, and it's really starting to bother me. Would lasers be helpful in removing the redness that I now have?"

Yes. Lasers for redness and broken blood vessels on the face have evolved remarkably over the last ten years. The older lasers, such as the original Candela pulsed dye laser (one of the first used for this problem), worked well but left large bruises that sometimes took several weeks to resolve.

The newer lasers work well *and* don't cause any bruising most of the time. Most patients now come into the office, have a treatment, put on makeup, and walk back out to normal activities. But be sure to check with your dermatologist about makeup because some doctors will restrict its use for a few days. They may also restrict or limit exercise for a few days to a week.

"What types of lasers are used to treat redness?"

There are a number of excellent lasers and intense pulsed light (IPL) devices used. The training, judgment, experience, and ethics of the doctor supervising or using the laser are more important than exactly which model of laser is used.

"Can I go right back to work after my treatment?"

Generally, yes. After most treatments, you may look like you have a light sunburn for a few hours or a day or two. Sometimes there's mild swelling for several days. The redness may be a little blotchy, but usually, foundation and concealer will cover this nicely, and you can go right back to your normal activities (except exercise). However, since recovery time varies, schedule your first treatment at the end of the day before a quiet evening. Then, once you know how you respond, you'll be more confident about what you can do after a treatment.

"Do the treatments hurt?"

Most patients tolerate the treatments easily. The lasers feel like a mild rubber-band snap against the skin. At my clinic, we have our patients pretreat themselves with

ELA-Max cream (lidocaine), a topical numbing agent that makes the treatment even more comfortable.

There's also a bright flash of light with the IPL devices—your eyes will be covered, but it can take a few minutes to get used to the light.

"How many treatments will I need?"

Usually, getting rid of most of the redness or dilated blood vessels will take three to eight treatments. If you have just a few small vessels, one to three treatments might suffice. If you're extremely red and have been so for many years, five to eight treatments might be needed. Ask your dermatologist for a rough estimate of how many you might need. Remember, though, if you engage in a lot of habits that induce frequent flushing (including *good* habits, such as exercise), you may need a few extra treatments.

"Are the results permanent?"

No. Nothing in the universe, including the effect of cosmetic treatments, is permanent. A common scenario is to need one or two maintenance treatments a year depending on how often you flush and blush; as well as on alcohol use, menopause, exercise, and many other individual variables.

"How much do laser treatments for redness cost?"

Costs vary according to the area being treated, where you live, and the skill of, and demand for, your particular dermatologist. A general ballpark figure for treating the whole face is $400 to $800 per treatment.

Nonprescription Creams

"Are there any nonprescription medicines I can use for my redness?"

The only nonprescription cream that's helpful at all for redness or rosacea is hydrocortisone, which comes in either .5-percent or 1-percent cream. This is a very mild anti-inflammatory cream in the steroid category. It does reduce redness somewhat, but it really doesn't address its root causes at all. While hydrocortisone cream may make the redness or rosacea look a bit less red temporarily, isn't nearly as good as those treatments available by prescription.

Using a little hydrocortisone cream while you're waiting to get in to see your doctor is probably fine. Just don't use it over long periods of time or in lieu of the better prescription treatments that are available. Almost all steroid creams can thin the skin if used incorrectly and can cause permanent dilation of blood vessels in the skin. Generally, hydrocortisone .5-percent and 1-percent aren't strong enough to do that unless you use them many times a day over a long period of time. (Don't use them for long around the eye area under any circumstance without first discussing it with your dermatologist.)

Propranolol and Clonidine

"I saw on the Web that there are medications that can be used to control flushing and blushing. Where can I find out more about these drugs?"

Several oral medications have been used for years with moderate success to help control flushing and blushing. Propranolol and clonidine are the two most commonly used. Because these are prescription drugs and they can have serious side effects, you'll want to make an appointment with your dermatologist to discuss them. You should also let your primary-care physician know that you're considering these medications, particularly if you have asthma, heart problems, or are taking a lot of other medications.

Summary of Redness: What to Do

Redness can stem from several different causes, but there are two main issues to be addressed: (1) How do you control or limit it? and (2) how do you get rid of the redness that you have? As with all issues that may involve a disease such as rosacea, check with your doctor or dermatologist to be sure you know what's happening in your case.

Here's what you should do to control or limit more redness:

- Use a good **sunscreen.**

- **Avoid triggers** for redness.

- **Understand the causes** of your redness, such as hormones in pregnancy or menopause.

- Get **treatment** for rosacea if you need it.

The treatment you receive from your doctor may very well control the appearance of the redness, but it probably won't eliminate what you had when you began treatment. Also, if you have rosacea, it's important to get it under control before seeking cosmetic treatments for the redness. You don't want to undo the progress you'll make by leaving the rosacea untreated.

For reducing redness, lasers are unquestionably the best option. They usually require a series of three to eight treatments, but they leave little or no bruising and usually require no downtime at all. The only real downside is the cost: Treating the face can run from $400 to $800 per treatment, depending on your doctor and where you live. But lasers work really well to diminish redness.

In the next chapter, we'll explore how to deal with blotchiness and under-eye circles.

ᕯᕲ ᕯᕲ ᕯᕲ   ᕯᕲ ᕯᕲ ᕯᕲ

7

BLOTCHINESS AND UNDER-EYE CIRCLES

It's a sad fact that no one over the age of 30 naturally has the smooth and even skin color of a child. As we get older, blotchiness and dark circles just come with the territory. Whether this discoloration stems from too much sun, skin diseases such as acne or rosacea, or reactions to products or medications, few things look worse cosmetically than a blotchy complexion.

Of course, the cosmetic industry can offer temporary cover-ups, but blotchiness is one area where modern dermatology offers some real help for the underlying discoloration. Lasers, in particular, are now so gentle that they can remove redness and broken blood vessels without breaking the skin. Let's take a closer look.

WHAT ARE THE POSSIBLE CAUSES?

- Acne
- Rosacea
- Seborrhea
- Perioral dermatitis
- Sun damage
- Picking
- Insomnia
- Skin-care products
- Medications

WHAT ARE THE POSSIBLE TREATMENTS?

- Bleaching creams
- Lasers
- Nonprescription remedies
- Sunscreen
- Antibiotics
- Lifestyle and product changes

POSSIBLE CAUSES

Acne

"It seems that whenever I have an acne breakout, it leaves behind red spots that last for months. What can I do about this?"

Acne causes inflammation in the skin, and the inflammation can create more damange than the acne itself. The inflammation causes new blood vessels to form and dilate as the skin tries to heal the acne lesion. And in many people, it also creates more pigment to deposit as an accidental by-product of the healing response. If you're lighter skinned and have a red undertone to your skin, your spots will likely be red after your acne heals; if your skin is darker, your spots will usually be brown.

Treatment. The most effective treatment is to prevent the problem altogether by controlling the acne. That's the first step. After you've done that, you can focus on getting rid of the spots. Make sure that you see your dermatologist if you've had moderate to severe acne for more than two months. She may treat you with creams, antibiotics, oral contraceptives, or even Accutane for the most severe acne. Deeper cystic acne lesions can be treated with an injection of a mild anti-inflammatory medication, which will make the lesion heal faster and decrease the chance that you'll get those blotchy red or brown spots or scarring.

If your post-acne spots tend to be brown, you might ask your dermatologist about a prescription-strength bleaching cream. Using 4-percent hydroquinone on the area during the breakout may prevent a dark spot from forming at all.

Rosacea

"I have rosacea. I've been using my medication faithfully for six months now. I don't have breakouts anymore, but I still have blotchy red discoloration across my cheeks. Why won't this go away?"

Your rosacea medication has probably improved the redness and decreased the pimple-like breakouts associated with it. But unfortunately, rosacea medication won't eliminate much of the redness and dilated blood vessels that have developed up to this point.

It's important to keep using the medication that your dermatologist prescribed to keep the rosacea under control and prevent its progression. But all of the blotchiness that was there when you started treatment may not disappear with medication.

Treatment. After your rosacea is under control with medication, the best treatment for the remaining blotchy redness is lasers.

Lasers can now eliminate most of that redness very safely and gently, with little downtime and without breaking the skin at all. Not only can lasers remove the little dilated blood vessels on the face, but they can also remove most of the permanent flush that may remain. And they're very gentle compared to the lasers that were used for this condition some years ago. However, a series of treatments is usually necessary. Ask your dermatologic laser surgeon for a recommendation.

Seborrhea

"Is there anything I can do about the red and scaly patches I have around my nose and eyebrow area?"

You most likely have a very common condition called *seborrhea*. This condition is usually characterized by red, scaly patches on the scalp, around the base of the nose, and sometimes in the eyebrow area. In severe cases, the redness and scaliness can extend down to the forehead, across the bridge of the nose, or even to the chest.

In the past, this condition was believed to be related to dryness, but now we know that isn't true. All of us have lots of microscopic organisms on our skin, including a tiny yeast form that lives in our hair follicles— and in the oil glands feeding the hair follicles—on our face and in our scalp. For reasons that aren't entirely clear, in some people this yeast overgrows and causes the scaliness you're describing. Similar to athlete's foot, there's probably a genetic susceptibility to this type of yeast.

Treatment. The first things to try are nonprescription remedies. Over-the-counter Nizoral A-D shampoo specifically controls yeast and has a dramatic effect on some patients. Try to use it daily. After you lather up your hair, put some of the shampoo on the affected areas, such as your eyebrows or the base of your nose (remember to keep your eyes closed so the shampoo won't irritate your eyes). Leave the shampoo on for about five minutes and then rinse it out well. The more often you wash your hair, the more the seborrhea will improve. Try alternating Nizoral with one or two other "dandruff" shampoos such as Sebulex, Head & Shoulders, or those shampoos containing zinc.

You can also try using a little bit of over-the-counter hydrocortisone cream (.5-percent or 1-percent). This is safe to use on the face, but if you have to use it every day to control the redness, you should see your dermatologist, who may prescribe prescription-strength Nizoral shampoo. There's also a prescription Nizoral cream that can help seborrhea around your nose or in the eyebrow area. You can try mixing the Nizoral cream with some one-percent hydrocortisone as well.

If the seborrhea is really stubborn, prescription oral medications such as Diflucan (fluconazole) may be used, but this is rare.

Perioral Dermatitis

"I get red bumps around my mouth and sometimes near my nose. My dermatologist says this is perioral dermatitis. What exactly is this?"

Doctors and researchers aren't quite sure what causes this annoying and unsightly condition. Some believe it's a relative of rosacea;

others think it's a type of bacteria or yeast. Soaps, lotions, or other skin-care products can sometimes aggravate this problem.

Beware of applying topical prescription steroids (stronger than one-percent hydrocortisone) to your face without the approval of your dermatologist. These may take the red out and give you the illusion of a quick fix, but the improvement is almost always temporary. In the long run, these steroid creams can actually aggravate the problem.

Treatment. Perioral dermatitis is usually treated like rosacea. Oral antibiotics such as minocycline are often given orally for one to three months. Cream antibiotics may be used as well (Akne-Mycin is currently popular and contains erythromycin). Your dermatologist may use other treatments that she prefers.

Get the Most Out of Your Prescriptions

1. *Use them.* You'd be surprised how many people pick their prescriptions up and then just let them sit in a drawer. They definitely won't do any good there!
2. Many prescription creams, gels, or lotions take eight to ten weeks to really work. Hang in there! You probably won't see much change in two weeks, especially with acne treatment.
3. Oral medications act faster, but if you have uncomfortable side effects such as bad gas, diarrhea, or stomachaches, you probably won't want to take the medicine for very long. Call your doctor to get something different.
4. Sometimes pharmacies and doctors make mistakes. If something doesn't seem right, be sure to double-check the medicine with the pharmacist.
5. When you see your dermatologist, take all of your prescription medications with you. That way, you'll know exactly what you have, and she can make sure you got the right prescription if there are any problems or you're not better.

Sun Damage

"I'm a redhead who's only 30 years old. Why do my face, neck, and chest areas already look so blotchy?"

What you're seeing is probably sun damage, which can show up as freckles and tiny red blood vessels. The whiter your skin, the more likely you are to freckle.

Melanin, the pigment in our skin that protects us from the sun's rays, is our own natural sunscreen. And even though redheads are born with beautiful skin, it just doesn't make much melanin. That's why most redheads don't tan; they just burn and freckle.

You can see freckling and sun damage in redheaded children sometimes as early as the toddler years. It's extremely important for children with red hair to be protected at all times with sunscreen, hats, and protective clothing. Redheads are in the highest risk group for melanoma, a potentially fatal type of skin cancer.

Sometimes freckling and "age spots" are mixed with tiny broken blood vessels that give the area a reddish, blotchy look as well. This reddish-brown blotchiness (called *poikiloderma*) is most often seen on the sides of the neck and on the upper chest. Areas of skin that have poikiloderma are also at higher risk for skin cancers.

Treatment. The good news is that there are now lots of effective ways to treat this type of sun damage. First of all, start using a sunscreen every day on your face, neck, and chest (particularly on those areas with poikiloderma). Be sure that the sunscreen has at least an SPF 15 or higher and that it contains zinc (4 to 7 percent) or Parsol 1789/avobenzone. Apply it liberally, because people commonly do not apply enough.

The second thing you can do is to see your dermatologist and get a prescription for Renova cream (tretinoin). Renova works well on the face but is usually too irritating for the neck and chest. For these areas, your dermatologist may recommend a vitamin-A derivative such as retinol, other less irritating skin-renewal products such as Kinerase (available in drugstores), or a gentle alpha- or beta-hydroxy acid. Used nightly, these products will gradually help the skin return to better health and appearance.

After the skin has been sun protected and treated with renewal creams for several months, then it might be time to investigate either gentle laser treatments or light chemical peels. Look for a dermatologist who does laser photorejuvenation, which works well for this problem and is gentle. Peels don't work quite as well for this problem because they're good at removing brown discoloration but not tiny, dilated blood vessels.

The visible signs of this type of sun damage can be removed almost completely with very little downtime and moderate expense. The blotchy brown spots, freckles, red spots, and blood vessels will gradually fade away—leaving smooth, clear skin.

Picking

"My doctor tells me that I need to stop picking at my face. Is it true that this just makes the problem worse?"

Absolutely! Not only does picking at your skin transfer bacteria from your hands to your face (which may result in a bacterial infection on top of the excoriated acne), but picking ruptures the pustule, whitehead, or blackhead down deeper into the skin, where it causes more inflammation and redness. Also, enough picking can actually cause or increase scarring from acne or other facial rashes.

Now, having said that, picking is also a human habit. Some people pick their cuticles; some pick at little spots in their scalp; and others pick at their faces. Since almost everyone picks something at some time in their life, picking really becomes more a matter of degree than anything else. To pick something occasionally is completely normal—to pick obsessively until you cause damage and scarring is not.

When the picking becomes obsessive (doing it almost every day) and damaging, it can be a part of what's called *obsessive-compulsive disorder* in psychological terms. In some cases, it can become so severe that patients create large ulcers that take months to heal and leave deep scars.

Treatment. If your picking is serious, please talk to your primary-care doctor or dermatologist about getting psychological help. Sometimes a deeper problem, such as depression or anxiety, is what's causing you to pick, and treatment may be needed. Learning some simple behavior-modification techniques from a psychologist who is familiar with this problem may be helpful.

If your picking is of the more mild variety, here are some remedies you might try:

- First, see if you can identify the time of day that you pick the most. Most regular pickers can point out a time that's particularly at risk for them, such as right before bed or after washing their faces in the morning. When you become aware of your most susceptible picking time, try posting sticky notes on the mirror to remind yourself not to pick.

- Try to substitute the picking behavior with another habit. For example, when you feel that overwhelming urge to pick, rub a little .5-percent hydrocortisone cream into the spot instead. That may give you the feeling that you're accomplishing something without actually picking at the lesion.

- Conceal the lesion with a cover-up pencil. Sometimes the temptation to pick becomes irresistible when the problem is staring you in the face, but if you can cover it up, you may be able to resist the impulse to pick at it.

- Keep in mind that a good aesthetician may be able to extract blackheads and whiteheads for you. You might want to make an appointment for a professional facial.

Insomnia

"I've been a little depressed for the last few months and have had trouble sleeping. Could this be why my skin is looking so blotchy?"

Yes. Insomnia can sometimes make your skin look unhealthy, because sleep allows your skin to repair itself in many ways. When you sleep, your skin mends itself from some of the damage caused by ultraviolet rays during the day. Your skin also rehydrates itself as the fluid that accumulates in your lower legs during the day re-equilibrates up toward your face and neck. In addition, blood supply to your head and neck increases as you lay down during the night.

If your skin is looking blotchy from lack of sleep, here are some suggestions to help you with your insomnia. If these don't work, be sure to seek medical attention, for you may be depressed or anxious. Also, if you haven't told your primary-care physician about your feelings of depression, please call today and make an appointment so that she can help you with that problem as well.

For insomnia, try the following:

- Go to bed at the same time each night if possible, and get up near the same time each morning.

- Get enough exercise. Don't work out close to bedtime, since the exercise-induced "high" could keep you from sleeping for several hours afterward.

- Closely monitor what you eat in the evenings: Too little food can sometimes cause low blood sugar and restless sleep in the early-morning hours, while too much food can make you sluggish. (Be aware that alcohol can interfere with your sleep cycle.)

- Avoid caffeine in tea, coffee, and colas, or large amounts of chocolate, after the noon hour.

- Make sure your mattress is a good, supportive one and that the temperature in your bedroom is comfortable.

- Try a warm bath, soothing music, lovemaking, or meditation before bedtime.

- Don't nap more than 15 or 20 minutes at a stretch, as this can interfere with nighttime sleep.

Skin-Care Products

"I recently bought a new skin-care regimen at a department store, and ever since I started it, my face seems to be all blotchy. Should I stop using these products?"

The answer to this is not as obvious as you might think. Some skincare products currently on the market are formulated in such a way that they *do* cause a small amount of irritation for a week or two in the beginning. It can be difficult to determine whether this is normal and will go away eventually, or if there's a problem with the products themselves.

It can be normal to have a little bit of pinkness and mild scaling for up to a week or two with a product containing vitamin-A derivatives, such as Renova, Retin-A, or tretinoin (the generic name); prescription acne products; or alpha-hydroxy acids or any other skin-rejuvenation product. If you're still getting the reaction after two weeks of use, stop the product and call your doctor to see if it's too harsh for your skin.

If, however, you're bright red and very irritated or have any blisters, yellow crusts, itching, or a burning sensation, you should stop using the product immediately and call your dermatologist. Yellow crusts, blisters, tenderness, pain, or the rapid spread of rash or fever can signal an infection or even shingles (*herpes zoster*), so you should see a doctor right away.

If the problem isn't so severe and you have to wait before seeing your dermatologist, try just using Cetaphil Gentle Skin Cleanser with Cetaphil cream or any other hypoallergenic cream. Try one-percent hydrocortisone cream several times a day to reduce the reaction. You should also take the product back to the cosmetic counter where you bought it. Most reputable companies will refund your money if you have an allergic reaction or a severe irritant reaction to a product.

After you're completely healed, don't start using your products all at once—if you have a reaction again, you won't know which one is causing it. Instead, add them back in one at a time, approximately three or four days apart, so you can determine which product is causing the problem.

Good Products for Sensitive Skin

Look for products that specify the word *hypoallergenic.* This means that they're less likely to cause allergies, but they aren't foolproof. Try the Free & Clear product line (**www.psico.com**) for products free of fragrances, most preservatives, lanolin, and formaldehyde. Other good products to check out are the Cetaphil line, the Eucerin line (but avoid this if you're lanolin sensitive), or Lubriderm.

Some of my patients have problems with most creams. If that's the case for you, try using just plain oils such as olive or safflower oil, or ask a good herbal apothecary to mix you a custom blend. (This will only work if you're dry—if you're acne prone, oils will just aggravate your condition.)

Medication

"I recently started taking a new medication for high blood pressure, and I've noticed that every time I go out in the sun I develop a red, blotchy rash on my face and other sun-exposed areas. Is this normal?"

Usually skin reactions to oral medications involve the whole body . . . but not always. There are some medications, such as those prescribed for high blood pressure, that can cause reactions *only* in sun-exposed areas. If you're taking a new medication and you also have a new blotchy rash on your face and/or other sun-exposed areas, be sure to talk to your physician about the medication.

Most reactions to oral medications will occur within several days to several months of starting the medication, but that's not set in stone. If you have a new rash and aren't sure what's causing it, be sure to bring your dermatologist a list of your medications and tell her when you started taking them. This can be very helpful in sorting out whether or not your rash is due to a new medication.

These reactions are generally treated by simply discontinuing or substituting a different medication, but that should only be done in consultation with the doctor who originally prescribed the medication. If the medication is critical and cannot be discontinued or substituted, your dermatologist can advise you and your doctor how to alleviate the reaction while continuing the medication. Sometimes rashes that occur in response to medicines will get better with time, even if the medication is continued.

Under-Eye Circles

"I get enough sleep, but I still have dark circles under my eyes. I've noticed that most people in my family do, too. What causes this?"

Under-eye circles are more complicated than you might think. Some are inherited—if that's the case, you'll notice them in other family members, too. Sometimes these inherited circles show a brown pigmentation around the entire eye rather than just underneath it. The brown discoloration often slowly increases with age.

Circles with more of a purplish or reddish undertone are caused by the superficial blood vessels in the skin showing more than they normally do. The skin around the eyes is very thin, so blood vessels show

through the skin more. These blood vessels tend to enlarge slightly as we get older; these types of circles also usually look worse with lack of sleep.

In addition, when you don't spend enough time lying down, fluid doesn't get a chance to re-equilibrate from your lower body to your upper body. The result is a hollow look around the eyes. That fluid redistribution is also responsible for puffiness in the eye area after a long night's sleep (especially as we get older), after too much salt intake, or from allergies.

As we age, the thin layer of fat that we have all over our face shrinks (atrophies) somewhat. As a result, the skin lays more directly over the muscles and blood vessels in the eye area. This can accentuate the darkness and sagging. Unfortunately, at this point in time, there are treatments that may help a little, but there's still no "miracle" cream or cure for under-eye circles. It's one of those problems we'd all like a quick fix for, but there's nothing that works consistantly yet.

Treatment. Obviously, getting enough sleep really helps. If you're consistently shorting yourself a half an hour to an hour a night, make a determined effort to get more sleep.

If you have the inherited type of brown pigmentation around the eyes, peels and lasers may work well for you. However, because the skin around the eye area is very delicate, it's sometimes better to do multiple lighter treatments than one deeper peel. If the area is reddish, vascular lasers to remove or shrink the small blood vessels that cause redness may be helpful. (Eye shields will be used to protect your eyes during treatment.)

Your dermatologist or dermatologic laser surgeon can advise you on the best option in your case.

Keep in mind that treating this area is a slow process and will require patience and a series of treatments. Expect improvement, but not complete resolution or perfection.

SUMMARY OF BLOTCHINESS: WHAT TO DO

Blotchiness can result from a number of different causes. The red, scaly patches of seborrhea may require Nizoral cream; the uneven redness of rosacea and perioral dermatitis may call for creams or oral antibiotics. Your dermatologist can diagnose your particular problem.

But let's suppose that the problem is not that easy to pin down. Here's what you should consider:

- One of your **skin-care products** could be causing the problem. You can become allergic to something even if you've used it for a long time.

- If you're taking a new oral **medication** (or even nonprescription drugs such as ibuprofen, herbal medicines, or vitamins), that could be the culprit.

- Drink less coffee, get more sleep, get rid of the junk food, and exercise a little—you'll be surprised how quickly these **lifestyle changes** will show up in your skin.

- **Don't pick** at your skin or overuse facial scrubs or loofahs. Treat your skin a little more gently—for healthy skin habits now will help you to have radiant skin throughout your life.

- If your blotchiness comes from sun damage, use a good **sunscreen** every day and talk to your dermatologist about tretinoin and gentle laser treatments. They can be very effective.

PART III

TEXTURE PROBLEMS

8

LUMPS
AND BUMPS

As we get older, a variety of lumps and bumps can make their annoying appearance on our faces. Sometimes moles that were once fairly small seem to grow bigger and have more hair; sometimes we notice a smaller version of those raised brownish spots that we saw on our grandfather's balding pate; sometimes acne flares up well past our adolescence; and sometimes we just notice growths that mar the texture of our face.

These lumps and bumps are usually benign, yet each kind of growth responds to a different treatment. Only your physician can tell you for sure what they are, but this chapter will at least provide you with a jumping-off point for dealing with lumps and bumps as you age.

WHAT ARE THE POSSIBLE CAUSES?

- Milia
- Enlarged oil glands
- Acne
- Moles
- Seborrheic keratoses
- Keratosis pilaris
- Fibrous papules of the nose

WHAT ARE THE POSSIBLE TREATMENTS?

- Topical creams
- Electrocautery
- Liquid nitrogen
- Microdermabrasion
- Light glycolic or salicylic acid peels
- Surgery

Possible Causes

Milia

"I have small, white, hard bumps on my face that are definitely not acne—I assume this is the case because they never go away. They last for months or even years. What are these, and how can I get rid of them?"

These bumps are called *milia,* and they're a type of very small cyst that hardens under the skin. And, as you obviously are aware, milia are very difficult to get rid of on your own.

If you try to squeeze or remove these bumps, this will usually cause so much trauma that your skin will look even worse. Your dermatologist, however, can remove these bumps easily with special tools. So if you have more than a few, it makes sense to make an appointment to get them taken care of professionally. Sometimes, if the bumps aren't too deep, a good aesthetician can remove them with a small lancet without too much trauma. If they're numerous, however, it may take several appointments to get rid of all of them. But make sure you don't have these bumps removed right before an important function or presentation, because you'll look a little marked up for approximately three to seven days.

Your dermatologist will probably make a tiny, almost invisible incision over the top of the bump and will then use a tool called a *comedone extractor* to pop the milia out. Afterwards, there may be a little crusting or blood around the area

for a day or two, or a bruise that may last up to a week or so, but people usually heal quite quickly from this treatment.

Also, creams in the vitamin-A family—such as Renova or Retin-A (tretinoin) or alpha-hydroxy cream—if used for a month or two before extraction, may help to loosen the milia a little bit and make them easier to remove. Renova or glycolic acids used over time may also help prevent milia from forming at all, so if you're someone who's prone to them, you may want to ask your dermatologist about a prescription for Renova (or another product if it gives you redness or peeling). Micro-dermabrasion can also help, because it sloughs off dead skin and cleans out the pores.

Enlarged Oil Glands

"I've had oily skin all my life, and now I'm noticing that I have very bumpy skin, too. The bumps don't seem to be acne because they don't move around at all. What are they, and what can I do about them?"

From what you're describing, it's very likely that these are enlarged oil glands, also called *sebaceous hyperplasia.* These show up as very small, soft bumps that are slightly yellowish or off-white in color. (It's best to have your dermatologist check to be sure, for small skin cancers can sometimes look similar.)

Unlike milia, these bumps aren't hard, and they tend to be the same texture as skin. Also, if you look very closely, you may see a small pore in the center of each bump—they're basically just oil glands that have enlarged over time.

Many of us have one or two of these bumps on the forehead, chin, or around the nose where most of our oil glands are concentrated. However, if you have very oily skin, along with large pores and acne problems, you may have a lot of the bumps. And while most people won't notice if you have a couple of bumps, if you accumulate quite a few, they'll give your skin a lumpy appearance.

Your dermatologist may recommend any number of treatments, but it's not advisable to have the bumps surgically removed and then sutured, because the resulting scars would look worse than the bumps themselves. In addition, microdermabrasion does *not* work very well for this, neither do the lighter peels performed by most aestheticians, such as glycolic or salicylic acid peels. CO_2 or erbium laser resurfacing will remove the bumps because these peels take off the entire top layer of skin and allows new "baby" skin to grow in. But it's definitely overkill for this problem—unless you have other issues such as acne scarring, a lot of wrinkling, or sun damage.

Electrocautery. My favorite method of treating enlarged oil glands is with a small electric instrument that looks like a pencil and essentially burns off the bumps. Electrocautery flattens the bump nicely and doesn't cause much redness. It leaves a small crust while it's healing, which heals in three to seven days depending on the size of the original spot. Usually the procedure can be done with no scarring at all.

The one disadvantage of this method is that sebaceous hyperplasia will eventually grow back. But it can take anywhere from several months to even years for that to happen. (If the bumps do reappear, they can just be flattened again.) Be aware that most insurance companies will consider this treatment cosmetic—which it is—and won't pay for it. The cost for doing this is usually in the $90 to $500 range depending on how many bumps you have.

Liquid nitrogen. Another possibility is to apply liquid nitrogen to the bumps to freeze them. This option takes longer to heal and causes more redness and irritation around the bumps than electrocautery. It may also scar occasionally.

Will It Hurt?

Most of us have had the experience of being in a doctor's office and having something done to us that we're not quite ready for. It's perfectly reasonable to ask your doctor, "Will this hurt?" and "Can any kind of anesthetic be used?" Here's a general description of how some of the procedures described in this chapter feel.

1. Liquid nitrogen elicits a mild to moderately uncomfortable burning sensation, and can be quite painful for warts on the palms and soles of the feet. The area treated might be sore for hours to days. Try taking acetaminophen or ibuprofen regularly for 24 hours before being treated.

2. Electrocautery uses what looks like a small electric pen (also called a *hyfercator*). The treatment is done very quickly in a short "zap" that feels hot. Any discomfort, however, tends to be gone quickly.

3. Opening up milia itself for extraction usually isn't felt, but if a comedone extractor is used afterwards, you'll feel a very short, mildly to moderately uncomfortable pressure sensation while the extractor presses on the skin for a few seconds. There's rarely any discomfort afterwards, but there may be a temporary small dent in the skin.

4. Surgery's only discomfort stems from the injected anesthetic, which varies from almost nothing with buffered lidocaine and a skilled nurse, to quite uncomfortable (unbuffered lidocaine and less skill). Your pain tolerance is also a factor. After the shot, there's no discomfort. Ask your dermatologist what to expect post-procedure, since this will depend on what you had done.

Acne

"I have dozens of tiny little bumps on my forehead and chin, with a few blackheads as well. What are the small bumps? Are they part of my acne?"

Yes. There are different types of acne and different treatments for it. From your description, you probably have *comedonal acne,* which is one of the most common types (the word *comedone* essentially means "plugged pore"). This kind of acne has an almost sandpapery texture, and consists primarily of blackheads (open comedones) and whiteheads that are little flesh-colored bumps covered by a thin layer of skin (closed comedones). Sometimes these tiny closed comedones can occur by the dozens on the forehead, nose, chin, and even sometimes on the cheeks.

Comedonal acne is usually not red. If these pimples do turn red (become inflamed) and form a head, then the acne is becoming more severe. You should see your dermatologist if this happens.

Although comedonal acne can be very annoying, it usually responds well to treatment. Prescription treatments work well for this type of acne, as can light glycolic acid or salicylic acid peels and microdermabrasion. Even going to an experienced, well-trained aesthetician may be beneficial: Your face may be steamed and the comedones gently extracted as part of a facial.

Microdermabrasion. A method by which very fine crystals are vacuumed across the skin under pressure with a tiny vacuum-cleaner-like tip, microdermabrasion works quite well for this type of acne. The fine crystals, coupled with the suction, take off a layer of dead skin, help clean out clogged pores, and improve circulation to the skin.

Depending on how many comedones you have and how sensitive your skin is, five to ten microdermabrasion treatments tend to be done one to two weeks apart. Then a maintenance program of a treatment every four to eight weeks may be recommended.

Light glycolic or salicylic acid peels. This is another option for treating comedonal acne. Like microdermabrasion, light chemical peels also take off a layer of dead skin, help clean out pores, and are used in a series. Low-strength acid is stroked onto the skin and left on for several minutes; the acid then either self-neutralizes or is neutralized by the nurse or aesthetician performing the treatment.

There are, however, occasional complications with light chemical peels if the aesthetician or nurse isn't experienced—this is particularly true for darker skin types. Sometimes the acid can be absorbed more in one spot than another and leave a temporary dark mark. Blisters can occasionally form, but scarring is rare. If you decide to go this route, find a dermatologist-supervised nurse, or an aesthetician experienced in performing these peels, particularly if you have darker skin.

Moles

"I have several moles on my face that seem to be getting larger and have hair growing out of them. Is it possible to remove them without leaving a big scar?"

Yes, it's usually quite easy to surgically remove moles. You'll always be trading the mole for a scar, but the question is: Is it a good trade? If the scar is barely visible and the mole is quite raised and noticeable, then you probably will think it's a good trade to have it removed. If the mole is tiny, it may not be such a benefit to have it done.

Your dermatologist can advise you on the best option for your particular mole(s). Most of the time, you don't need a plastic surgeon to remove a mole unless it's in a particularly bad spot. And keep in mind that insurance companies tend to view cosmetic mole removal as medically unnecessary; therefore, they won't cover it. But most dermatologists charge a reasonable fee for this service.

Surgery. There are two ways to remove the moles you're describing. The most common method is to numb the skin and take the top of the mole (the colored part) off, leaving the base of it in place. Usually that leaves an almost invisible or barely noticeable scar when it heals. Even if there is a slight color difference between that area and the surrounding skin, it can usually easily be covered with makeup.

Healing usually takes one to two weeks, and the area may remain slightly reddish or brownish for several months afterwards. If injuries to your skin tend to take a long time to heal completely, it's likely that your skin may be pink or brownish for several months after removal of the mole. The color, however, will almost always return to normal eventually.

It's important to keep the site moist with an antibiotic ointment (or whatever else your dermatologist recommends) during the healing time; it can also be kept covered with a bandage if you want. Have your dermatologist instruct you on wound care, as post-procedure infections, while very uncommon, *can* occur.

There's one caveat for removing the mole this way, however: It could grow back in the future. Pregnancy, in particular, sometimes stimulates moles to grow, or they'll just grow on their own for no particular reason. If that happens, the same procedure can just be repeated, with an excellent cosmetic result.

The only other disadvantage to this method is that hair follicles aren't removed, so if the hair growing out of the mole really bothers you, you should consider this next method. (By the way, it's fine to tweeze hair out of moles. It's strictly an old wives' tale that doing so is harmful.)

The second method involves removing the entire mole. Your dermatologist will take a small cookie-cutter-like instrument approximately the same size as the mole, and remove the entire thing, root and all. The wound is then closed with stitches. (The skin is numbed with a small amount of injected lidocaine before the procedure.)

The advantage of this is that the *entire* mole will disappear and will probably not recur; in addition, the hair follicles are removed. The disadvantage of this method is that it may leave a more obvious scar, depending somewhat on where the mole is.

If you decide to go with this method, the stitches usually come out in five to seven days, and the site itself can take weeks to months before it goes back to its natural skin color. Surgical scars can take a full year before they reach their final appearance, but most of the improvement will occur in the first three to six months.

Seborrheic Keratoses

"I have a number of small, brownish, dry, rough patches on my face and around my hairline. They're raised from the skin a little and almost look like warts. What are these, and what can I do about them?"

They're most likely a very common benign growth called *seborrheic keratoses.* Almost everyone over the age of 40 has at least a few of them somewhere, and they can occur anywhere on the scalp, face, trunk, arms, or legs. There's no evidence that these "barnacles" are caused by frequent hair coloring.

Seborrheic keratoses tend to have a slightly waxy, warty, raised, or "stuck-on" appearance. They often grow slowly, and can become quite large over many years. The "barnacles" can range in color from flesh color to very dark brown or even almost black depending on your underlying skin color. If you have dark hair and eyes, the growths are more likely to be a darker brown; if you have light hair and eyes, the growths are more likely to be flesh colored or light tan in color.

Seborrheic keratoses aren't skin

cancers, although if you're not sure about something on your skin, be sure to have your dermatologist look at it. Until a medical professional checks it out, it's very dangerous to assume that a new growth isn't cancerous. Also keep in mind that cosmetic removal of these growths generally isn't covered by your insurance company (unless the growths are irritated), but most dermatology offices now charge a very reasonable fee to have them removed.

Liquid nitrogen. This is the most common method for removing seborrheic keratoses. Liquid nitrogen is extremely cold and is stored in airtight, insulated cans. It's either sprayed on with a nozzle attached to a small handheld canister or applied with a cotton-tipped applicator for a variable amount of time depending on the thickness of the growths. Even though it's cold, when liquid nitrogen is applied, there's a burning sensation that can be uncomfortable depending on how long it needs to be applied to the skin. Afterwards, there may be a burning or throbbing sensation for a few hours or even days—take acetaminophen or ibuprofen if you're experiencing discomfort.

After the treatment, the site will usually get red and irritated around the base, almost like an insect bite, and then crust over or even occasionally blister a little bit. The most noticeable crusting or blistering is usually gone in two to four weeks. The site usually heals nicely over time, but may leave a temporary mark for several months after removal.

Keratosis Pilaris

"I've had red, scaly bumps on the backs of my arms, and sometimes on my face and thighs, for many years. My doctor said that this is inherited and there's nothing that can treat it. Is that true?"

The name for this problem is *keratosis pilaris*. It's indeed a genetic trait—if you ask around in your family, I'm sure you'll find someone else who has it, too.

This problem is caused by excess production of a protein called *keratin* that helps make up the skin cells that line the hair follicles. When keratin accumulates, it causes a plug to form in the hair follicle, which irritates the follicle and turns it red.

The reddish bumps appear most commonly on the back of the arms, but they can also show up on the thighs, buttocks, and other areas. Nothing can change the genetic makeup of your skin or "cure" this problem, but new skincare technology can help improve it. You should also try wearing looser clothing. The tighter your clothes, the more rubbing there is, and rubbing makes this condition worse, which is why symptoms tend to improve in the summer.

Topical creams. Retin-A or Renova and alpha-hydroxy acids may help dissolve the keratin plugs in the hair follicles, leaving the skin with a smoother, softer appearance. Also, mixing those products with over-the-counter hydrocortisone one-percent cream will often make the bumps appear less red. Try AmLactin or Lac-Hydrin cream, both of which can be purchased in drugstores.

If that doesn't work, your dermatologist can give you a specially mixed solution to try. I'll sometimes have a compound of salicylic acid, urea, and hydrocortisone mixed at the pharmacy for my patients. While there's no true "cure" for keratosis pilaris, this compound does tend to make the skin softer and less red. Your dermatologist may know of some other remedies for you to try.

Also, some of my patients think essential fatty acid supplements have helped them, but this is anecdotal. Trying them isn't harmful.

Fibrous Papules of the Nose

"I'm 35 and have a new firm bump on the tip of my nose. What is this?"

It's probably a *fibrous papule* of the nose. These are very common and benign. However, it's important to have this checked by a dermatologist, since certain skin cancers can look very similar. If it *is* a benign fibrous papule of the nose, it can often be removed or flattened by shaving or burning it off. Again, your dermatologist can advise you.

If there's any question that your bump might be a skin cancer, it will be biopsied. This is fine, since it removes the lesion and also allows the pathologist to examine the tissue.

SUMMARY OF LUMPS AND BUMPS: WHAT TO DO

No one treatment works for all the lumps and bumps that crop up on our faces as we get older. And, in fact, there's no real "high-tech" technique for treating any of these growths, partly because the standard methods still work pretty well.

Your best bet is to have your dermatologist look at any suspicious texture problems, because you want to be sure that you don't have skin cancer. Once a diagnosis is made, then you can decide what treatment is best for your goals—and your pocketbook.

෧෧ ෧෧ ෧෧   ෧෧ ෧෧ ෧෧

9

TOO OILY
OR TOO DRY

The next problem to tackle is skin that's too oily or too dry. You may not think of this as a texture problem, but oily skin often goes hand-in-hand with large pores, and dry skin often gets flaky or rough and bumpy.

Many things can affect the oiliness or dryness of your skin: Climate, hormones, and your genes can all play a role. Unfortunately, there are no high-tech treatments that eliminate oily or dry skin, but you can do a lot to improve your skin with the right information and care. This chapter will provide you with some in-depth knowledge about cleansers and moisturizers so that you can help combat your oily or dry skin.

WHAT ARE THE POSSIBLE CAUSES?

- Heredity
- Climate
- Menstrual cycles
- Oral contraceptives
- Hormone-replacement therapy (HRT)
- Large pores

WHAT ARE THE POSSIBLE TREATMENTS?

- Soaps and cleansers
- Toners and drying agents
- Moisturizers
- Makeup
- Microdermabrasion
- Lasers

POSSIBLE CAUSES

Heredity

"My mother has extremely oily, acne-prone skin, and mine seems to be developing that way, too. Is there a link?"

Yes, definitely. Most of us can trace our skin type directly to a parent or relative in our extended family. You see, we don't just inherit eye and hair color and basic skin tone from our parents—we inherit our oil glands from them, too. If you take after your mother's side of the family in other ways, chances are that you've inherited her oily, acne-prone skin as well. In fact, most patients who have severe cystic-scarring acne have a parent or other close relative who had the same condition.

Oil production in skin also increases dramatically at puberty. It continues through the 20s and then gradually decreases, particularly for women in their 40s and 50s as menopause grows near. This isn't always the case, however—some people have extremely oily skin well into their 50s, but it's quite rare for people in their 60s to have it. (The pattern in men is similar: oily in the teens and 20s, with a gradual decrease in oil into middle age.)

If you care about having good skin, you should try to be aware, as early as possible, what your skin type is. That way, you can start young and take measures to keep your skin well hydrated if you tend to be dry; if you're oily, there are a number of ways to keep pore size smaller and acne under control.

Climate

"I recently moved to New York from Palm Springs, and I've noticed that my skin has changed a lot. What effect does climate have on skin?"

It has a huge effect. Dry skin loves humid, open-air climates with moderate temperatures. If you have dry skin, you may have noticed that your skin problems improve within days of vacationing in Mexico, the Caribbean, or Hawaii. And dry places such as the desert or high mountain areas (and even long airplane trips) can make your skin feel as dry as a reptile's.

Conversely, oily skin likes drier climates—even though your skin's oil production is the same, it will feel drier because more moisture is evaporating off through the skin. Oily skin feels even more oily in moist, warm climates, since humidity prevents moisture from evaporating off the skin. In addition, oil helps hold water in the outer layers of the skin so that it can't evaporate.

But remember that climate isn't just related to the weather outdoors. Most of us work and live in buildings or dwellings that are heated in winter and air-conditioned in the summer, so these indoor climates become the most important ones as far as our skin is concerned. I see a noticeable increase in complaints about dry skin in Seattle (where I live) when the central heating comes on in the fall. The irony is that even though the climate outdoors is moist, many people spend the vast majority of their days in centrally heated indoor environments.

Normal or combination skin tends to be a bit more forgiving, but the T-zone area of the forehead, nose, and chin is slightly oilier in everyone and may seem annoyingly so in a more humid climate. The area around the eyes, neck, and sometimes cheeks is drier in everyone and may need extra moisturizing, even if you have an oily T-zone.

Menstrual Cycles

"I've noticed that my skin seems oilier at certain times of the month. Could my period have something to do with it?"

Most definitely. Oil production is closely linked to hormones, which fluctuate during menstrual cycles. During puberty, hormones bounce up and down quite a bit as menstrual cycles are being established—particularly if your periods are irregular. However, even if you have stable menstrual periods, estrogen or progesterone levels vary depending on that particular month's cycle. Also, some months we ovulate two eggs, in which case hormone production changes even more.

Many women notice an increase in breakouts and oil the week or so before their period, which correlates with a rise in progesterone levels. The approximate 28-day cycle for estrogen and progesterone goes something like this: Day one of your menstrual cycle is the first day you start menstruating. Bleeding usually continues for three to seven days, during which time estrogen levels slowly rise. Estrogen levels continue to rise until about day 14 (or midcycle), when ovulation occurs. The ovary that released the egg then produces progesterone. This progesterone production continues from approximately day 14 through about day 28, gradually increasing and then falling until menstruation starts again.

In some women, the cycle is longer or shorter but still regular. In others, the cycle is quite irregular, making it difficult to predict exactly where estrogen and progesterone levels are at any given time. And all women produce low levels of "male" hormones such as testosterone. These hormones are called *androgens,* and they also contribute to oily skin and acne. Women who have a condition known as *polycystic ovary syndrome* produce increased androgens and experience more problems with oily skin, acne, irregular periods, and increased hair growth on the face and sometimes other parts of the body.

Oral Contraceptives

"I recently went off the Pill, and I've noticed that my skin seems much oilier and more prone to breakouts now. Could the two be related?"

Yes. Many women report that birth-control pills improve their skin. Hormones control oil production, and since your hormones change within each menstrual cycle (and also from cycle to cycle), any medication that stabilizes your hormones, such as birth-control pills, may improve your skin.

All oral contraceptives will stabilize menstrual cycles by giving you a consistent amount of estrogen-like and progesterone-like compounds throughout the month. Just stabilizing the hormones may help reduce oily skin and acne. Also, some oral contraceptives are formulated particularly to help acne—for example, Ortho Tri-Cyclin was the first oral contraceptive approved by the FDA to treat acne *and* also act as a birth-control agent. In some women, oral contraceptives by themselves are enough to control oily skin and any acne that might be related to it.

It takes several months after starting oral contraceptives to see an improvement in one's skin. Conversely, once you've stopped taking them, it often takes several months for your skin to revert back to its natural baseline state. Remember that the health risks related to taking oral contraceptives increase after age 35 and if you smoke. Be sure to discuss any of these issues with the doctor prescribing your oral contraceptive. Give her your complete reproductive background and tell her if you or anyone in your family has a history of blood clots.

Hormone-Replacement Therapy (HRT)

"I'm going through menopause, and after thoroughly discussing the risks and benefits with my doctor, I decided to go on hormone-replacement therapy. But now my skin is oilier and breaks out sometimes—could this be related to the hormone replacement?"

It very likely is. Remember that oily skin and the acne that sometimes accompanies it are related to hormones, regardless of the source. So, if you're adding hormones back through hormone-replacement therapy (HRT), it can indeed cause breakouts.

As you know, HRT is a complicated issue. It sounds as if you've weighed all the different risks and benefits carefully with your primary-care physician, so please remember that the effects of HRT on skin are really secondary compared to its effects on heart disease, breast cancer, uterine cancer, and other serious medical conditions. To me, it doesn't seem appropriate to prescribe or not prescribe HRT just for skin problems.

Most HRT is a combination of estrogen and estrogen-like compounds, progesterones, and sometimes testosterone or other androgens. The most common regimens call for daily estrogen with progesterone cycling for the last ten days of the month, at which time a period occurs; or progesterone and estrogen given together consistently throughout the month so that a period doesn't occur. Progesterone helps keep the cells lining the uterus mature so they don't become cancerous. In the early days of HRT, only estrogen was given, and researchers found that that stimulated the lining of the uterus so much that cells could become cancerous more easily.

Usually low-dose estrogen alone isn't a problem as far as skin is concerned. It does seem to increase oil production slightly, but since most of us are significantly drier when we're about 50 anyway, the increased oiliness at that age can be a positive effect. The problem seems to come with progesterone and androgens. Most women who are taking progesterone for ten days or so out of the month notice that while they're on progesterone, they experience increased oiliness and acne breakouts, in addition to other symptoms of premenstrual syndrome (PMS). Testosterone has long been known to aggravate acne, and hormone-replacement regimens that include testosterone can aggravate oiliness and acne as well.

If you're having problems with your skin while on HRT, the best thing to do is to talk to both your primary-care physician and your dermatologist. Primary-care physicians are very knowledgeable about most aspects of HRT, but not all understand what HRT can do to the skin. Your dermatologist should be able to help you with your breakouts.

It may be possible to change the type of estrogen or progesterone in your HRT to one that doesn't cause as many breakouts. There are a number of different forms of progesterone, and many hormone-replacement regimens are different. If one type of progesterone seems to be causing a problem, it's often worth trying a different one to see if that particular form of progesterone is better for your skin. Progesterone can be taken in very small doses daily (rather than a ten-day course) in a combined estrogen/progesterone pill, which may alleviate oiliness and associated acne.

Another option is a new progesterone IUD that can be implanted directly in the uterus. It can deliver progesterone directly to the lining of the uterus where it's needed, without all of the systemic side effects of progesterone (oily skin, acne, and PMS-like symptoms such as mood swings). But be aware that insurance will often not cover these IUDs, and they can be expensive, so you should ask about cost first.

Large Pores

"What can I do about my large pores?"

We can land a man on the moon, but I'm sorry to say that nobody's figured out how to cure large pores yet.

Pore size is decided by a combination of the skin type you inherited from your family, the amount of oil your skin produces, whether or not you have acne or other skin diseases, and other factors that we don't know much about yet. Everyone's pores are generally larger on the nose and sometimes through the forehead and chin (the T-zone area) partly because those areas are oilier. But no matter what the factors are that contribute to large pores, most of us would love to be able to get rid of them.

Just trying to reduce your pore size isn't enough of a reason to go on medications such as Accutane or oral contraceptives—I simply cannot emphasize this enough. But if you need these drugs for any other reason, then you may discover that they do decrease your pore size a bit as they're decreasing your oil production. (A medication called *spironolactone,* which reduces testosterone levels a little, may also help.) This effect is usually temporary, since oil production will increase again as soon as you go off the medication.

Let's look at some other options.

Makeup. If you just want to cover up your pores, then this is a viable option. I've found that it's a mistake to use heavy makeup to cover large pores because it tends to pool in the pores after a few hours, which only accentuates them. If you use a foundation, try to find one that's light, has a sunscreen in it, and contains some light diffusers that will help make the skin look more even. One that I particularly like is Lancôme Maqui-Libre, which has all of the above-mentioned items. (Other cosmetic companies make excellent ones as well.)

It also helps to apply a light dusting of powder—many now even have light diffusers in them. It's better to apply powder with a brush than with sponge pads because pads tend to pick up too much powder, and they're more likely to harbor bacteria. Brushes can be cleaned well with warm water and shampoo once a week, and you can use either pressed or loose powder with them.

Makeup, of course, is only temporary, and what most of us really want is a permanent solution. Unfortunately, no "breakthrough" treatment has been proven to cure large pores, but here are some treatments that may help:

Microdermabrasion. Manufacturers of these machines often claim in their literature that microdermabrasion can decrease pore size, but there's never been any scientific data to prove this claim. And this is a difficult thing to prove or disprove since pores are so small. It's possible that over time and with multiple treatments, microdermabrasion might help reduce pore size, but so far there's no evidence to support this. However, many people with oily skin do find that their skin feels smoother and has fewer blackheads and whiteheads, even if their pore size doesn't change. Microdermabrasion may help to keep oil (sebum) and dead-skin cells from building up in pores.

Photorejuvenation. This is a series of gentle laser treatments that helps reduce the signs of sun damage and stimulates collagen production; this process has also been reported to decrease pore size. Improvement in pore size has been mentioned in both research studies and laser manufacturers' literature, and it's been subjectively observed by those of us who work with lasers every day. In my experience, many patients seem to notice a modest improvement in their pore size, but I think the jury is still out on this issue. The problem is that not everyone seems to receive that benefit, and it's very difficult to document small changes in the size of pores. In addition, when change does occur, it's really not known if it's permanent or temporary. I recommend that you undertake a series of photorejuvenation treatments for other reasons (such as sun damage, redness, dilated blood vessels, or early fine wrinkling); if your pore size happens to change in the process, you'll be pleased with the added benefit. However, you may be disappointed if you receive photorejuvenation treatments for large pores alone.

Laser resurfacing. Deep CO_2 peels or erbium laser resurfacing leave the skin much smoother and, as a result, may help to diminish the appearance of large pores. But because these lasers involve more risk and a long recovery period, they're *not* used for large pores alone. If you have a lot of deep wrinkles or acne scarring, laser resurfacing may be appropriate, and may have the positive side effect of improving the appearance of your pores.

POSSIBLE TREATMENTS

Soaps and Cleansers

"What kind of soap should I be using?"

Soaps and cleansers are confusing because there are so many of them, and so many different claims are made about them. Here's the bottom line: As long as what you're using isn't overly drying your skin, any soap or cleanser that's only on your skin for about 15 seconds isn't going to make a huge amount of difference.

There are three major types of cleansers: soaps, synthetic detergents, and lipid-free cleansing lotions. Let's look at each of them.

Soaps. Soap is made by mixing fatty acids with an alkaline substance, so soaps have what's called an *alkaline pH* (greater than 7.0). Some researchers feel that this alkaline pH has an undesirable effect on the skin. Transparent soaps contain glycerin, which helps counteract the drying effect. Super-fatted soaps contain a greater amount of lipids (fats) to provide a protective film on the skin. Deodorant soaps contain topical antibacterial agents that may help fight odor.

People with dry skin should generally avoid soaps, as their cleansing power and higher pH often strip the skin of moisture. For people with oily skin, soaps may be fine—it's a myth that oily skin just gets oilier if you wash it. Oil secretion is tied mostly to hormones and genetic skin type.

Examples of soaps are: Ivory soap (pH 10.1); Neutrogena Original Formula glycerin soap (pH 9.6); and Basis super-fatted soap (pH 10.6).

Synthetic detergents. Synthetic detergents are just cleansers made of human-made ingredients instead of fats from Mother Nature. All synthetic detergents contain agents called *surfactants,* which help break up oil, dead skin cells, and dirt on the skin, and carry them off in the washing process. Synthetic detergents, unlike soaps, have a *neutral* or *slightly acidic pH,* and some researchers feel that cleansing agents with this type of pH are less irritating for dry skin.

But the confusing thing is that many products calling themselves "soaps" are in fact synthetic detergents. Dove soap, for example, is a synthetic detergent that has a neutral pH (7.3). Some antibacterial "soaps," such as Lever 2000, are also synthetic detergents. Other examples include Aveeno Moisturizing Bar for dry skin (pH 4.9), and Cetaphil Gentle Cleansing Bar (pH 6.3–6.5).

Like soaps, synthetic detergents are probably best used if you have oily, normal, or combination skin. Despite the more favorable pH factor, synthetic detergents can dry out the skin too much for those with a tendency toward dryness (unless you get the Aveeno bar for dry skin).

Lipid-free cleansing lotions. Most of us with drier skin are using fat-free soaps, or lipid-free cleansing lotions, which are especially designed for people with sensitive or dry skin. These types of cleansers also leave less facial residue than classic soaps, which is another factor that can affect the irritation and drying potential of a cleansing agent. Some examples of lipid-free cleansers are Cetaphil Gentle Skin Cleanser (pH 6.3–6.5) and Purpose Gentle Cleansing Wash.

Some of these lipid-free cleansing lotions are even specially formulated for patients with oily skin who are occasionally also sensitive, or for combination skin. Examples of cleansers in this category would be Cetaphil or many of the cleansing, products now sold in dermatologists' offices.

What Cleanser Should I Use?

Like breakfast cereals, there are hundreds of different cleansers on the market. How do you pick one? The key issue is to avoid any cleanser that's overly drying. After that, it may come down to which one feels and smells the best to you—after all, it's only on your face for about 30 seconds twice a day. Here are several to try.

1. *For dry skin:* Try Cetaphil Gentle Skin Cleanser (sold in drugstores), M.D. Forté Facial Cleanser I (found in dermatologists' offices), Olay Foaming Face Wash and Purpose Gentle Cleansing Wash (sold in drugstores), and SkinCeuticals Foaming Cleanser (found in dermatologists' offices).

2. *For normal/combination skin:* Try Cetaphil Gentle Skin Cleanser (sold in drugstores) or M.D. Forté Facial Cleanser I (found in dermatologists' offices).

3. *For oily skin:* Try M.D. Forté Glycare Cleansing Gel for Oily Skin with glycolic acid (found in dermatologists' offices), any drugstore acne cleanser that has 5 percent or more benzoyl peroxide in it, or cleansers with salicylic acid.

Toners and Drying Agents

"Is there anything I can use to dry up the excess oil on my face?"

It would be wonderful if there really was something that could be put on the skin in the morning that would sop up excess oil all day long—unfortunately, we're still waiting for it. But here are some things that may help in the meantime.

Drying soaps. It seems logical that drying soaps would work well for this problem, but in fact, they seem to dry out the area around the eyes, neck, and cheeks too much while sometimes offering only marginal benefit in the oily areas. These soaps may reduce oiliness for an hour or two, but the effects are temporary and don't address what's driving the oil production: hormones and genes.

Toners and drying agents. Try Clinac O.C. (oil-control) gel, which is now available at pharmacies (you may need to ask them to order it for you). Various claims have also been made about toners to help with oily skin—many of them are alcohol based, but some aren't. Again, they may have a temporary effect for an hour or two, but they won't last much longer than that.

Makeup. It's important if you're oily or acne prone to stick with oil-free foundation, since you certainly wouldn't want to add any more oil. Some oil-free foundations have tiny particles in them that may help to absorb oil, while some are completely water based and might be a good option. Loose powder applied with a brush or pad will also absorb oil and reduce shine.

Blotting. One of the best things to try is the old-fashioned method of blotting. Take clean tissue paper and just blot it against the skin several times a day, allowing it to absorb the excess oil. This is better then overloading your skin with too much powder, and it's one way to absorb oil without actually having to take makeup off. MAC cosmetics (found at many department stores) sell a small packet of very fine blotting papers. Also try Clean & Clear Oil-Absorbing Sheets (available at drugstores).

Extra washing. If you're extremely oily, you might want to consider washing your face again around lunchtime. You can then reapply oil-free foundation and some light powder. Doing so may absorb oil through the end of the workday.

Moisturizers

"There are so many different types of moisturizers out there that I'm completely confused. What should I use and why?"

Moisturizers do two important things: (1) They add water to the skin; and (2) they help inhibit evaporation of water. Water in the skin is what keeps it "hydrated." Fats (often called *lipids*) are also important, as they help bind water to the skin and hold it there. When the level of moisture (hydration) in the outer layer of the skin falls below a certain level, the skin feels dry, stiff, sometimes flaky, or cracked. Moisturizers essentially bind water to this outer layer of skin so that it feels moist, supple, and smooth. The three main types of moisturizers are creams, lotions, and gels.

When you look at the label of a moisturizer, it's very difficult to know what type or quality of moisturizer it is—or even what half its terms mean. For instance, *emulsion* means that the ingredients are all mixed up together so that they won't separate. (When you beat an egg, you emulsify it.) To make matters even more confusing, moisturizers are now often combined with other products such as sunscreens and skin-rejuvenation ingredients such as vitamins or alpha-hydroxy acids.

The quality of the moisturizer depends partly on its basic ingredients and also on how it's all put together. The more expensive moisturizers tend to hold water in the skin better, but they're also what's called *cosmetically elegant.* This just means that they absorb into the skin more easily, are smoother, and have a nicer feel and fragrance than some of the inexpensive ones do. Generally speaking, higher-quality moisturizers do hydrate the skin and maintain hydration better than inexpensive ones.

For your body. Moisturizers that dermatologists often recommend for general use all over the body include Cetaphil Moisturizing Cream, Vanicream, Eucerin Original Moisturizing Creme or Lotion, Keri, Lubriderm, and Curel. All of these, especially if applied right after a bath or shower on damp skin, will help keep your skin hydrated. Applying these moisturizers daily or even twice a day is par-

ticularly important if you have any skin diseases, such as atopic dermatitis or psoriasis.

Some dermatologists' offices now sell body moisturizers that contain 10 to 15 percent alpha-hydroxy acid. These body lotions not only hydrate the outer layer of the skin, but the alpha-hydroxy acids exfoliate dead skin cells a bit better than plain moisturizers.

There are some excellent over-the-counter moisturizers that contain ammonium lactate, which has a similar effect as alpha-hydroxy acids. Two of these products are AmLactin and LacHydrin 5-percent lotion. LacHydrin is also available by prescription at a higher concentration. Products sold at drugstores and dermatologists' offices tend to be better quality and more affordable than similar products sold in department stores. But if you still like the one that has your favorite fragrance in it, you'll have to buy it at a department store.

For your face, neck, and chest. The trend in facial moisturizers now is to maximize therapeutic effects while moisturizing. You may see many different therapeutic vitamins added to moisturizers now, but there's no evidence that piling as many of these on as possible does anything except possibly irritate your skin. Almost all of the renewal agents now on the market were studied as single agents and not in combination. Plus, using two or three rejuvenation products at a time may dilute the effects of all of them, or the combination may have negative effects that we don't understand—we really don't know at this point. What follows is a summary of the different therapeutic vitamins that you might see added to moisturizers now.

Vitamin-A derivatives are prescription medications such as Renova (tretinoin) and over-the-counter derivatives such as retinol. Retinol is converted by an enzyme in your skin to tretinoin; since you have a limited amount of that enzyme, using retinol is like using a weak form of tretinoin. Tretinoin increases dermal collagen production, normalizes abnormal sun-damaged skin cells *(keratinocytes)*, helps exfoliate the outer dead layer *(stratum corneum)* of cells, and increases cell turnover rates. The very largest body of scientific data support its use, while the data for retinol is much less.

Alpha- and beta-hydroxy are sometimes referred to as "fruit acids" because they're derived from natural sources such as sugar cane, grapes, and milk. They include glycolic acid, which is derived from sugar cane and is probably the best known of these acids. The effects are similar to vitamin-A derivatives, and a significant body of data supports their use.

Vitamin C helps prevent the damage that ultraviolet light does to skin by protecting the skin's own immune system, but *it is not a sunscreen.* It may stimulate collagen growth and help normalize sun-damaged skin. There is a moderate body of data to support its use.

Vitamin E may augment the action of vitamin C and may act to help protect the skin's own immune system from damage from UV radiation, but there's not much data from studies with humans to substantiate this claim.

What Should I Be Putting on My Face?

Feeling confused about the zillions of moisturizers and skin-rejuvenation products out there? Here is a simple and rational approach to get you started. If you have easily irritated skin or skin diseases such as rosacea, don't try these without seeing your dermatologist first.

1. *Morning.* Wash with a cleanser, and apply a moisturizer with a sunscreen containing zinc or Parsol 1789 in it, such as SkinCeuticals Sun Defense SPF 20 (found in dermatologists' offices) or Cetaphil Daily Facial Moisturizer SPF 15 (sold in drugstores), to your face, neck, and chest. Use an eye cream around your eyes—try Dermalogica Total Eye Cream SPF 15 (available in salons), Cetaphil cream (sold in drugstores), SkinCeuticals Primacy Eye Balm Vitamin C Eye Gel, or M.D. Forté Replenishing Eye Cream (found in dermatologists' offices).

2. *Night.* Wash with the same cleanser. Start with one renewal product such as Renova (if you can tolerate it) or M.D. Forté I cream. Use just the one product for two to three months—if you're doing well with that,

try alternating nights with a second product, such as a good topical vitamin-C solution like SkinCeuticals C & E (found in dermatologists' offices) or an alpha-hydroxy product if you're using Renova. Use an eye cream, just as in step one.

If you want to try adding in more products, talk to your dermatologist first. And, if you're very dry, you may need an extra moisturizer. Try M.D. Forté Replenish Hydrating Cream, SkinCeuticals B5 Moisture Enhancing Gel, or Emollience (found in dermatologists' offices). Drugstores carry Cetaphil Moisturizing Lotion (or Cream) or Neutrogena Visibly Firm Night Cream, both of which work very well, too.

If you really want to take advantage of some of the therapeutic agents that are proven to help reverse sun damage and improve the quality of skin, try the basic program outlined in this chapter. Then talk to a dermatologist who has an active cosmetic practice. She can advise you on which therapeutic products aimed at skin rejuvenation and reversing sun damage might be helpful for you.

Remember, be sure that the dermatologist with whom you make an appointment has a cosmetic practice, because some dermatologists only practice medical dermatology. So check before you schedule an appointment. If a good dermatologist isn't available in your area, try to find the most knowledgeable aesthetician that you can. She may be able to make good product recommendations.

10

TREATING SCARS

We all have scars somewhere on our bodies, but the ones on our faces seem to bother us the most. Whether they stem from acne, a childhood fall, a traffic accident, or a basketball game, scars may be cherished parts of our personal history . . . or constant reminders of a particularly painful experience.

What can we do about scars? Do lasers hold some promise for getting rid of them? And what are the techniques for treating them? This chapter will answer these questions and more.

WHAT ARE THE TYPES OF SCARS?

- Acne scars
- Keloids, and hypertrophic scars
- Surgical scars
- Accident-related scars

WHAT ARE THE POSSIBLE TREATMENTS?

- Injections
- Reexcision
- Punch grafting
- Subscision
- Collagen
- Paper tape and silicone
- Dermabrasion
- Chemical peels
- Lasers and laser resurfacing

THE TYPES OF SCARS

Acne Scars

"I developed acne several years ago. Could the scars I'm seeing on my face now be from that?"

This is actually a more complicated question than you might think. Many types of acne leave a red or brownish mark on the skin after the lesion heals—these are temporary (they usually go away in two to six months) and aren't true acne scars. Many patients are confused when I tell them this, so allow me to explain.

True acne scarring is a *permanent* depression, elevation, or white area on the skin, which follows cystic acne (hard, tender, deep lesions) or very inflamed pustular acne (plugged pores with pus in them). The texture of this type of scar tends to be firmer than the surrounding skin.

There are also different types of acne scars. For example, one type, called an *ice-pick scar,* leaves a deep pit with a narrow opening at the skin, as if a tiny ice pick had punctured the skin. Other acne scars affect the surface of the skin and can have either rolling soft shoulders or sharply demarcated, almost perpendicular, boxlike walls. Still other types of acne scarring may look like very enlarged pores where the acne was active.

The recommended treatment varies according to the type and amount of scarring you have. The most common treatments for acne scarring are simple excision, subsci-sion, punch grafting, CO_2 and erbium laser resurfacing, dermabrasion, and collagen. I'll discuss all of these later in the chapter.

Keloids, and Hypertrophic Scars

"I recently had a mole removed from the middle of my chest. It now looks worse than it did before and is hard, raised, and sometimes painful and itchy. Can I get this scar removed?"

What you've described sounds like a *keloid,* or *hypertrophic scar.* (Let's just call them *keloids* since the treatment is usually the same for both.) Keloids are scars that become raised, firm, painful, and/or itchy instead of staying flat and soft through the healing process. Keloid formation often begins four to eight weeks after mole removal but can happen later as well—they can also occur after any type of skin injury or in response to skin diseases where there's a lot of inflammation, such as acne.

Keloids can crop up just about anywhere on the body, but they're most common on the chest, over the shoulders and upper back, and at sites of piercing, particularly the ears. Keloids are also age related. The risk for them jumps at puberty (around 12 or 13) and gradually increases through the late teens and early 20s. The risk starts to decrease again in the 30s, but a few unlucky individuals are prone to keloids their entire lives.

It's important to tell your doctors (particularly surgeons) if you're keloid prone, because keloids caught early are much easier to treat than ones that have been present for a long time. With special surgical techniques and injections, they can sometimes even be prevented after surgery. Once they've developed fully and have matured, keloids can be quite difficult to treat and may require multiple visits to the doctor to get and keep them under control. Common treatments include injections of potent anti-inflammatory drugs into the scar, reexcising and then trying to prevent reccurrence, laser treatments, and using tape or silicone gel on the scar.

Surgical Scars

"I've had a number of surgeries over the years, and the scars have always healed well. I had shoulder surgery about six months ago, and the scar is ugly and very large. Why hasn't it healed as well as the others have?"

The way scars heal depends on a whole host of factors, but generally, the more tension there is on the scar while it's healing, the worse it will look. For example, scars around the eyelids heal very nicely because there's usually extra skin in the area, thus causing very little tension on the scar. Similarly, caesarean section scars right above the pubic bone also often heal well because there's extra skin after delivery and almost no tension on the scar.

But scars over a joint, such as the shoulder, get a lot of tension. The joint, the skin, and the scar move frequently, and the skin is often pulled somewhat tightly over the joint. While a scar on the abdomen may heal into a nice, neat white line, a scar over a shoulder or a knee can spread and look quite wide. And the more heavily muscled a person is, the more stretch the scar gets. Sites at high risk for unsightly scars are the chest area, the joints, and the back, particularly in people whose job requires lifting.

Interestingly enough, age can work to our advantage in this area. When we're older, our skin is looser and less elastic, so there's less tension on wounds, which results in smaller, less obtrusive scars. Conversely, in younger people there's a lot of skin elasticity, which places more tension on wounds and tends to make scars spread more.

Almost all surgeons do what they can to minimize the spreading of scars by putting in absorbable stitches down in deep layers of the skin where they can't be seen. This relieves tension on the wound by reinforcing the layers of skin under the surface. These deep sutures support the skin while it's healing after the superficial stitches are taken out, and can last anywhere from 4 to 12 weeks. In addition, your surgeon may ask you to limit your activity and wear surgical tape or Steri-Strips (a special type of post-surgical tape) over the scar for many months to help keep the scar flat, soft, and narrow.

What Are Stretch Marks?

Stretch marks are a special kind of scar that arise from inside the skin rather than from a tear or incision on the surface. When skin is asked to stretch too far too quickly, collagen and elastic fibers that hold the deeper layers of skin together rupture and create a deep tear but no surface tear.

Stretch marks most commonly show up on the abdomen in pregnancy, especially if a woman is carrying twins or triplets. But they're also common in teenagers during growth spurts, particularly over joints such as the shoulders (in boys) or over the hips (in girls). Rapid weight gain in adulthood can cause them, too.

There's no cure yet for stretch marks, nor is there any hard evidence to support the claim that massaging in vitamin E oil or other creams will help. There have been some reports that certain lasers, microdermabrasion and/or Retin-A may help, but these haven't been confirmed in studies involving large numbers of people. If the marks stay red, lasers can help normalize the color, but red stretch marks usually fade with time on their own without any treatment.

Accident-Related Scars

"I was recently in a terrible car accident and was left with several unsightly scars. My doctor said I should wait at least six months to a year before I consider having these treated. Why is that?"

Scars attain only about 60 percent of their final wound strength at about six to eight weeks after surgery; they then continue to remodel silently under the surface of the skin for up to a year—which is why many doctors recommend waiting. But it never hurts to get a second opinion from another doctor.

Since stitches usually come out of wounds at one to two weeks, good surgeons will often reinforce a scar for weeks to months afterwards by using Steri-Strips or surgical paper tape that you can buy at the drugstore. Reinforcing the wound by keeping the scar tightly closed and as flat as possible maximizes your chances of a smaller scar. And the scar's appearance will gradually improve over time without your having to do anything about it. Your own body's healing mechanisms are really quite amazing.

If after six months to a year the scar is still quite red, raised, or irregular in some other way, then it may be time to visit your dermatologist and consider some of the options discussed in the next section.

(The exception to this is development of a possible keloid. If after six to eight weeks or longer, the scar becomes itchy, painful, or more raised, be sure to have your doctor look at it.)

POSSIBLE TREATMENTS

Injections

"My doctor recommended scar injection for me. What exactly is this, and what does it do?"

Doctors have used scar injection for many years to reduce keloids, which form when the normal wound-healing response goes awry. The cells in the wound that make collagen don't stop when the wound is flat with the skin. Instead, they keep producing collagen until the scar is raised and hard—and often itchy and painful as well. In addition, inflammatory cells and extra blood vessels may collect around or in the scar and make the area look red. To help combat this, your dermatologist will inject a strong anti-inflammatory medication directly into the scar, usually in a series of injections three to four weeks apart. The medication (usually triamcinolone) turns off the cells producing the excess collagen and causing the inflammation. Thus, the scar slowly gets flatter, softer, and less itchy and painful.

The needles used for these injections are often so tiny that they cause very little discomfort. However, since the scar itself is often already inflamed and painful, just injecting fluid into an area that's already sore may cause a fair amount of discomfort. As the scar gets softer and less inflamed over time, the injections will become more comfortable. (This treatment is usually covered by medical insurance.)

Reexcision

"Several years ago, I had a mole removed from my back. The scar has spread a lot and looks quite unsightly. Is there anything that could improve it?"

If it's flat and soft but just wide, sometimes reexcising it may be a good solution. When a scar is reexcised, your dermatologic surgeon goes back through the exact same area of the original scar, cutting out the scar tissue and restitching the incision.

Your surgeon will put extra-reinforcing absorbable sutures deep in the layers of the skin to help hold the wound together. Paper tape or Steri-Strips may be used on the scar for several months to help keep the scar from spreading.

You may also be asked to refrain from exercise, which stretches the scar as well. If you exercise regularly, be sure to discuss any restrictions with your surgeon—there's no point in undergoing a scar reexcision only to undo the benefits by going back to bench presses or rowing too soon after the surgery.

Some acne scars can be treated with excision as well. This works best on acne scars that have a narrow opening but are deep ("ice-pick" scars). A tool that looks like a round cookie cutter and comes in a number of different sizes can be used to excise the entire scar, and then one or two tiny stitches are put in to hold the new edges together to make the skin surface smooth and flat. After the stitches have come out and the area heals, it may look fine on its own. However, if it still needs some work, a chemical or laser peel may improve the appearance of the area even more. This can be done in conjunction with punch grafting (discussed below).

Punch Grafting

"I have a lot of acne scarring, and my doctor recommended punch grafting and excisions. Could you explain what this is?"

Punch grafting starts with the procedure discussed above. First, the scar is excised with a small circular tool just slightly larger than the scar. Then a little piece of skin is taken from another site on the body, often from behind the ear. That piece is then placed into the hole where the acne scar once was. Occasionally this will be stitched into place, but often it is just held with some surgical tape or even just allowed to heal on its own, with the pressure of the surrounding skin holding it in place. The small area behind the ear from which the grafted skin was taken is then stitched together with fine sutures.

The small plug of skin that was put into the scar can sometimes heal in such a way that it's raised a tiny bit above the normal plane of the skin. This can be dealt with in several ways. It can be sanded down with special tools used for dermabrasion, making the scar flat with the skin. Laser resurfacing or dermabrasion might then be done over the entire face, including the new little punch grafts, to make the texture of your skin smooth and even. Different dermatologists have different preferences in this regard, but the resulting improvement is significant. (Keep in mind, though, that only certain types of acne scars can be treated with this method. Your dermatologist may not recommend this at all if you don't have the type of scarring that responds well to this treatment.)

Is Acne Scarring Preventable Now?

Yes, for the most part it is. If the acne causing the scars (usually cystic or pustular acne) is caught early and treated with a course of Accutane, oral antibiotics and/or oral contraceptives and topical agents, it's now possible to stop scarring acne in its tracks before it becomes permanent and widespread.

If you have any signs that your acne might be starting to scar, see your dermatologist as quickly as possible to get started on treatment. If conservative treatment isn't working after two or three months, consider Accutane. Or, if your acne is severe enough, it may even be appropriate to *start* with Accutane.

Subscision

"My acne scars are more shallow, broad depressions in my face rather than deep holes. My doctor has mentioned scar subscision. What is this?"

First, your doctor is on the right track in discussing scar subscision with you, because this process works best for shallow scars with a broad base (such as yours), rather than the deeper "ice-pick" scars that we discussed previously.

To understand scar subscision, you need to understand how you got your scars in the first place. The depressions in your skin developed because the acne lesion disrupted the normal formation of collagen under your skin as it healed. The collagen didn't form in a normal, smooth, wavy layer running parallel to the surface of your skin; instead, it bunched up into a thick bundle that permanently pulled down the surface of your skin.

During scar subscision, your doctor will numb the area first and then push a small needle through the skin down to the area where the collagen is all bunched up. She'll then work the needle around to break up that abnormal collagen layer, and a small pocket will often fill with blood under the scar. As the area heals, the new collagen formation will push the scar's base up a little.

It usually takes anywhere from one to four treatments, depending on how deep the scar is, to lift the scar area up close to level with the skin surface. You'll probably see small improvements after each treatment. The only downside to this technique is the bruise that's left right after the procedure, which tends to last one to two weeks and is annoying—but it can usually be covered with makeup while the area is healing. The time between treatments is generally 4 to 12 weeks.

After you've had as much improvement as you can get with the subscision, you may want to consider laser resurfacing, dermabrasion, or a medium-depth TCA peel to even out the skin's surface even more.

Collagen

"My dermatologist recommended collagen for my acne scars. Do you have an opinion on this?"

Collagen injections work quite nicely for shallow, broad-based acne scars, but they don't work well at all for deep scars with a narrow opening. If you have the former type, the only downside to collagen is that it's temporary and has to be repeated approximately every two to six months, depending on how long it lasts on you as an individual and what area of your face is being injected. Also remember that it's very important to be allergy tested twice before undertaking any collagen treatment.

Collagen is used less now for acne scars than it used to be, because the treatment modalities mentioned above are more permanent.

Paper Tape and Silicone

"A friend told me that silicone sheets would be helpful in improving one of my scars. Is this true?"

There's been a lot of marketing in the last few years regarding the use of silicone-based products to improve scars. These sometimes come in the form of sheets that you cut into a shape to fit the scar and leave on for varying periods of time. There's also a silicone gel called *Mederma* that you can rub into scars once or twice a day to soften them and improve the appearance.

Several studies have shown that scars did indeed improve after several months of using these silicone-based products. But a recent study comparing these products to plain old paper surgical tape showed no significant difference between the paper tape and the silicone products.

It turns out that what seems to matter most is simply covering the scar. Just putting something over a scar to inhibit evaporation of moisture through the skin over weeks to months appears to soften, flatten, and improve the appearance of the scar. Bear in mind that fresh scars are far more likely to show improvement than scars that have been there for years.

For years, many surgeons have recommended the use of Steri-Strips or just plain flesh-colored paper surgical tape over scars to reinforce wounds and improve their appearance during the healing period. You can easily get surgical paper tape from the pharmacy and try it instead of the silicone sheeting. It's best if the tape can be worn 24 hours a day for a period of several months.

If the scar is in a covered part of the body, you can just leave the paper tape on and shower and do all your normal activities until it falls off on its own. There's no need to take it on and off every day, for if you do, chances are that your skin will get irritated from the tape itself. Also, you may be allergic to tape, so if you get red and itchy, take it off immediately. And if you don't like it, then by all means try the silicone products.

Dermabrasion

"My dermatologist recommended that my acne scars be treated with dermabrasion. What's the difference between this and laser resurfacing?"

Laser resurfacing has largely supplanted dermabrasion in the last ten years, but dermabrasion is still an excellent procedure in the hands of a skilled physician.

Dermabrasion can be done on the entire face or just a section. The area is numbed well, usually with a local anesthetic. The tool itself looks a little bit like a drill, except instead of a drill bit there's a small, smooth wheel that comes in various shapes and sizes. This wheel, which is covered with a very fine diamond dust, is used to sand down through the skin in a very controlled manner in order to remove the acne scars. Dermabrasion is a very bloody procedure, which is another reason it isn't done as much anymore—it's highly risky to operating-room personnel if the patient has Hepatitis B or C, or is HIV-positive.

With dermabrasion, almost more than any other dermatologic procedure, it's extremely important to find someone with lots of training and experience. Most dermatologists who are highly skilled in dermabrasion now are over 50 years of age. Many of the younger dermatologists, including myself, didn't receive training or have a lot of experience with it because we started out using lasers.

Chemical Peels

"I asked my dermatologist if a chemical peel would help my acne scarring, and she said that it wouldn't. Why not?"

Unless you have very mild, very superficial acne scarring, chances are that a trichloroacetic acid (TCA) peel won't make much difference. It's difficult with even a deep TCA peel to get enough depth to make much of a difference with acne scarring or to fine-tune TCA for different spots on the face. Some parts absorb the chemical more than others, and some areas of acne scarring would need a deeper peel than others. This can be challenging to calibrate with a chemical peel.

With a laser resurfacing or dermabrasion procedure, on the other hand, most of the face can be lightly lasered or dermabraded. Then the area with the worst acne scarring can be treated to a greater depth and greater precision to ensure maximum improvement.

Laser Resurfacing

"What are the different types of lasers used for resurfacing acne scarring, and how do they work?"

The carbon dioxide (CO_2) laser and the erbium YAG (Er:YAG) are the two main lasers used for resurfacing as a treatment for acne scarring. These lasers have largely supplanted dermabrasion and chemical peels, because in experienced hands they yield results comparable or better than dermabrasion, with less bleeding and fewer risks. (Be sure to find a dermatologist who has a laser center and is very experienced with this procedure.)

With both lasers, tiny micron-width layers of skin are removed until the laser surgeon reaches a level that will have the best effect on the acne scars without risking complications. This is both a science and an art and takes considerable experience to do really well. Good laser surgeons can pretty much tell exactly what depth they're working in by the appearance of the skin and as a result of their experience on different parts of the face. For example, skin over the nose is much thicker than skin right around the jawline. The laser surgeon will adjust the depth according to the part of the face being worked on and the depth of the scarring itself.

Laser resurfacing may be recommended by itself for certain types of acne scarring or may be combined with a number of other procedures discussed above, including excision, punch grafting, or subscision. In fact, CO_2 laser resurfacing can be performed after or at the same time the other procedures are being done.

Lasers

"I have a red keloid that has only partially improved with injections. My doctor recommended using a laser for this. What do you think?"

There's a lot of data now to support the use of vascular lasers, which are used to treat dilated blood vessels, remove redness, and help shrink keloids and hypertrophic scars. Vascular lasers can be used to treat scars that have been healed for six months or more but are still red. The lasers help take the red out very nicely.

These lasers are safe, with generally no downtime associated with them. The scar may look slightly redder for a couple of days after the procedure or maybe even bruise temporarily. Multiple treatments are necessary to achieve good results, and they're often done in conjunction with (or in between) triamcinolone injections.

Laser procedures for treating scars are effective, but they're also expensive. Treatments run anywhere from $200 to $500 or more per treatment depending on where you live and the size of the scar to be treated. This can get quite expensive if you need three to ten treatments to make a difference, especially since insurance companies don't tend to pay for it, as they consider it cosmetic.

SUMMARY OF SCARS: WHAT TO DO

The treatment of a scar depends on what type you have, so your doctor will have to see it to advise you on possible treatments.

The traditional treatments—injection, reexcision, punch grafting, and subscisions—all have good track records and can work well depending on your scar and the skill of your doctor. Lasers, while expensive, can bring about excellent improvement in red scars and some other types of scars. And laser resurfacing can really help with certain kinds of acne scars. The bottom line: See your dermatologist and be sure to find an experienced laser practitioner.

ೲ ೲ ೲ   ೲ ೲ ೲ

11

DEALING WITH UNWANTED HAIR

So much of beauty is really just fashion. Take hair: Having facial and body hair is perfectly normal—just about every woman has some. Europeans have no problem with this. In fact, women in France and Germany usually don't shave their legs or their armpits.

But American fashion calls for smooth, hairless women (and sometimes men), so most of us in North America have resigned ourselves to preventing hair from intruding in certain places on our bodies. The most striking development in this area is the use of lasers, which make it possible to dramatically reduce the amount and texture of unwanted hair. Whether it's embarrassing hair on a young woman, new hair appearing after menopause, or hair on a back or neck that a man wants gone, lasers can bring welcome relief.

WHAT ARE THE POSSIBLE CAUSES?

- Your family
- Polycystic ovary syndrome
- Hormones
- Medications

WHAT ARE THE POSSIBLE TREATMENTS?

- "Physical" hair removal
- Electrolysis
- Vaniqa cream
- Laser hair removal and maintenance

UNDERSTANDING NORMAL HAIR GROWTH

"Why does hair grow more in some areas of the face and body than others?"

We human beings are born with hair follicles all over our bodies, probably courtesy of our primate ancestry. Babies are covered with fine, soft down called *vellus hairs,* but as we grow older, hair follicles in different parts of the body produce thicker, longer hairs. The triggers for this change are hormones.

Even in childhood, boys usually have more hair—which tends to be longer, darker, and slightly coarser—on their arms and legs than girls do. And as puberty approaches, boys' hairs get signals from hormones to start growing, particularly in areas such as the armpits, the genitals, and the beard. As hormones diminish in middle age, hair growth gradually recedes in many areas, and pubic hair gets lighter in density, as does hair on the head.

As for baldness, hair on men's heads doesn't just fall out, contrary to popular belief. Rather, the hair follicle itself gradually gets smaller and smaller, and the hair finer and finer, until at last there's just a miniature hair in the place of what used to be a long, dark, coarser one. This is generally referred to as *male-pattern baldness.* Women can also experience this kind of thinning (and even baldness), particularly if there's a history of men and women on both sides of the family with this kind of hair loss.

Hair also has a growth cycle. All hairs go through a growth phase, a resting phase, and a falling-out phase, after which new hair growth begins again. This hair-recycling time varies in different parts of the body. For instance, hair on the face grows faster than on other parts of the body; thus, its growth cycle is shorter—so, if you want to have the hair on your face treated with a laser, the treatment interval will often be approximately four weeks. In contrast, the hair-growth cycle for other parts of the body is from eight to twelve weeks (depending on the body site), so you may be asked to return for treatments at longer intervals.

Most of us seeking hair removal are concerned about the coarser, longer, darker hairs that grow where they're not wanted. But soft, fine, vellous hairs can sometimes be a problem as well. Certain medications in particular can cause these blonde hairs to become quite thick and begin to look like "peach fuzz." A new hair-growth inhibitor called *Vaniqa cream* may help, since vellous hairs don't respond well to laser reduction.

Research is quite active in the area of hair development and biochemistry, since drug companies haven't missed the fact that men will pay huge amounts of money to cure their baldness. However, many aspects of hair texture, quality, and growth are still mysterious: The hormones and genetics of hair development have turned out to be far more complicated than anyone would have thought.

WHAT ARE THE POSSIBLE CAUSES OF UNWANTED HAIR?

Your Family

"Many of the women in my family have a lot of facial hair. Is that something I'm likely to develop, too?"

Yes. There's definitely a family resemblance in hair-growth patterns: In some families, many women have fairly long, coarse, dark hair on the arms; on the chin and sideburn area; and sometimes around the nipples and on the abdomen. If this is something that runs in your family, don't worry—it's perfectly normal. If you wish, your unwanted hair can be removed with lasers (discussed later in the chapter).

It's extremely rare, but increased hair growth occasionally does indicate other serious endocrine-gland imbalances. Usually this type of hair growth is associated with severe treatment-resistant acne. Again, discuss this with your doctor if you're concerned, for blood tests can confirm or deny your suspicions.

Polycystic Ovary Syndrome

"My doctor thinks I may have polycystic ovary syndrome and says that this may be the cause of my increased hair growth. Can you explain?"

This disease (which may be hereditary) causes the ovaries to be full of small, fluid-filled sacs, or cysts, which interfere with the production of normal eggs.

Many women with polycystic ovary syndrome have some difficulty getting pregnant and tend to have acne and increased hair growth due to more circulating "male" hormones. Hair may be slightly thicker all over the body, but it's generally most noticeable on the face and in the abdominal area. The hair can be very stubborn and require more laser treatments than average to remove it and keep it under control.

Polycystic ovary syndrome is also associated with acne. A medication called *spironolactone* may be helpful in lowering testosterone levels enough to help keep the hair and acne under better control. Oral contraceptives may also be helpful in regulating your period and hormone levels.

Hormones

"I'm in my early 50s and going through menopause. Why am I suddenly developing dark, coarse hairs on my chin and upper lip?"

The increase in facial hair is just one sign of a hormonal change going on all over your body. During menopause, hair on the chin, upper lip, and sometimes the abdomen starts to increase in thickness and length, while hair in the temple area starts to shrink. Since you now have fewer circulating female hormones, hair in the armpit and pubic area will get sparser, too.

All women have both female and so-called male hormones: Our female hormones are predominantly estrogen and progesterone, and our "male" hormones are primarily testosterone and DHEA (dihydroepiandosterone). In menstruating women, levels of estrogen and progesterone fluctuate all month long in a predictable pattern that results in a monthly period, and the effects of these hormones in your monthly cycles override some of the effects of male hormones.

Approaching menopause, however, estrogen and progesterone levels drop because periods are starting to become less regular and ovulation doesn't occur every month. Thus, there are more male hormones (also called *androgens*) present relative to female hormones. And these androgens cause the changes in hair follicles that you've noticed.

Medications

"I recently began taking a new medication, and I think I'm starting to grow more hair on my face. Is this possible?"

Yes. Many medications can affect hair growth or loss, and some can even cause both growth *and* loss because they have different effects on different people.

Some of the most common medications that make hair grow more are prednisone, Dilantin, and other anti-seizure medications, tamoxifen (sometimes used for breast-cancer treatment), and testosterone. There are also many others, so if you think a medication may be aggravating hair growth, be sure to discuss this with your primary-care physician or dermatologist.

The list of medications that can make hair fall out is even longer—but if hair loss does occur due to medication, it's almost always temporary. Some of the most common offenders are medications for blood pressure (such as atenolol) and Accutane (a medication used for acne for which hair loss is a mild and temporary side effect). But there are dozens of others—if you're concerned, check with your doctor.

POSSIBLE TREATMENTS

"Physical" Hair Removal

"What's the best way to remove hair without spending a lot of money?"

The so-called physical methods of hair removal are still very effective and inexpensive. Their only real disadvantages are that they're temporary and sometimes painful.

Plucking. The belief that plucking hair will make it grow back thicker and coarser is an old wives' tale—hair doesn't grow back differently just because you plucked it. It's also fine to pluck hair out of moles.

The benefit to plucking (and waxing, too) is that it lasts longer than shaving and hair-removal creams because you're removing the hair at its root rather than just cutting it off at the surface of the skin. When you pluck, make sure that you have adequate lighting and good-quality tweezers. Clean the tweezers with an alcohol wipe before and after each treatment so that you don't collect unwanted bacteria on them.

If you're planning to have laser hair-removal treatments done, be sure to let the hair grow back in for at least four to six weeks before the treatment. The laser beam won't be able to find the hair to zap it if it isn't present in the hair follicle.

Waxing. Waxing is also an excellent method of hair removal—when done by an experienced and licensed aesthetician. A thin layer of warm wax will be applied to the area and allowed to harden for a minute or so. The wax is then quickly pulled off the skin, taking the hair and a thin layer of dead skin with it. Be sure to let your aesthetician know if you're using vitamin A or its relatives (Retin-A, Renova, tretinoin, Differin, Tazorac, retinol, and so on), as your skin may be more fragile or sensitive. Waxing will generally last about two to three weeks on the face and three to five weeks on the legs depending on how fast your hair grows.

Waxing rarely transfers infections, because the wax is usually kept fairly hot. But some women have trouble with irritation and ingrown hairs afterwards. If you tend to get irritated, applying one-percent hydrocortisone cream (available in drugstores) to the area once or twice a day for a few days after the waxing should alleviate some of the irritation. However, if you have a lot of problems with ingrown hairs after waxing, you may want to opt for laser hair reduction and maintenance.

Shaving. This is probably the most common hair-removal method used by American women. To minimize irritation, be sure to shave in the bath or shower after the hair has been warm and wet for at least five minutes. Shaving creams also help, as opposed to soap, because most of these creams are formulated to soften hair better.

If you don't use disposable razors, be sure to change your blade at least weekly so that you don't collect bacteria that might infect your hair follicles. If you get mildly irritated or have a few ingrown hairs after shaving, try one-percent hydrocortisone cream on the area for a few days. If you have a lot of trouble with ingrown hairs after shaving, you may want to opt for laser hair reduction and maintenance instead. Also, shaving spreads flat warts, so if you have those on your legs, don't use shaving as your method of hair removal—you may end up with warts all over your legs. (Waxing is fine while the warts are being treated.)

Hair-removal creams. These aren't as popular as they once were, mainly because the strong chemicals that break down hair tend to really irritate the skin surrounding the hair as well. Some women can use these creams successfully, but many find that they're too irritating, particularly over the long haul. Like shaving, hair-removal creams are temporary because they remove the hair from the skin surface rather than from the root of the follicle.

Electrolysis

"In what situations would you recommend electrolysis for hair removal? Isn't it less effective than laser hair removal?"

Electrolysis is actually very similar to laser hair removal in its effectiveness. However, since each follicle must be treated, electrolysis is a slow process and best for small areas. Each individual hair follicle receives an electrical current that's passed down a tiny wire into the follicle—which is usually more painful than laser hair removal.

Electrolysis may still make sense if you have only small areas of hair that you need to have removed, such as on your chin or upper lip. As with laser hair reduction and maintenance, one treatment won't take care of all of the hair, and multiple treatments are usually required. Infections and scarring may be complications of electrolysis, so be sure to look for a licensed, experienced electrolysist. It's helpful if they have a medical background, but it isn't absolutely necessary. Your dermatologist may know of a good one in your area.

Vaniqa Cream

"I've recently seen Vaniqa cream advertised in commercials. What is this, and how does it work?"

This relatively new cream is an excellent choice if you have a limited amount of hair in an area such as your chin, or if your hair is blonde or gray. Also try it if you have lots of blonde "peach-fuzz" on your cheeks, for laser hair removal does not work very well on blonde or gray hair yet.

Vaniqa is usually rubbed into the area to be treated twice a day, and it's also relatively inexpensive. However, since it works by inhibiting the growth of the hair but does not kill the root, if you stop using the cream, the hair will grow back.

Laser Hair Removal and Maintenance

"How does laser hair removal work?"

The laser emits a very specific beam of light targeted at melanin, which is the pigment in our hair and skin that gives it color. Laser hair removal is easiest when the hair is dark and the skin is light because all of the laser beam energy is then absorbed by the hair and not by the skin. But with certain types of lasers tuned just right, dark hair on dark skin can be removed, too. It just needs to be done with extra care and may take more treatments.

"Why does the hair grow back?"

Remember that hair grows in three stages—growth, resting, and falling out. The laser won't destroy hairs in their resting phase, so you have to come back at intervals to make sure that all the hairs get treated during their growth phase. The next treatment can be done as soon as additional hair growth appears.

Any single treatment may injure the hair bulb (the source of the hair) but not kill it. The effects of the treatments are cumulative over time: Lasers gradually reduce the number of hairs that grow back, but the hair will also become lighter and finer in texture as the treatments progress. On average, three to seven treatments are necessary to achieve the best results, but certain parts of the body require fewer treatments because the hair cycles through its phases more slowly.

"Who should be doing laser hair removal?"

There's a lot of controversy right now about who should do laser hair removal. Currently, each state regulates laser hair-removal systems as it sees fit. In many states, only physicians, physicians' assistants, or registered nurses (RNs) supervised by a physician may perform this treatment; in others, aestheticians are allowed to own and operate laser systems.

The problem is that serious complications, including permanent scarring and discoloration, can occur from a laser treatment gone wrong. For that reason, my personal opinion is that only dermatologists, their supervised physicians' assistants (known as *PACs*—who receive a higher level of training than an RN), or RNs should do laser hair removal.

Some clinics claim to have a physician on staff, but they're rarely actually on-site. This, in my opinion, does not constitute physi-cian supervision—I believe the doctor should do more than just check in occasionally from an off-site office.

The bottom line is patient safety, and laser hair-removal systems are safest in the hands of dermatologists, who are physicians that specialize in the care of skin, hair, and nails. Laser hair reduction performed by someone not medically trained or supervised may be cheaper, but you have to balance the cost with the risks. I think your safety and appearance are reasons not to scrimp on laser hair reduction.

"How long does the treatment last?"

Many people report that after three to seven treatments their expectations have been met and the hair-growth pattern is much, much less. However, you can expect to need more treatments if you have any history of irregular periods, polycystic ovary syndrome, or family history of excessive hair. In addition, maintenance treatments may be recommended.

In some areas of the body, the laser will not only decrease the number of hairs but will make the hairs very fine and lighter in color. Not all of the hairs will be permanently eradicated, but the decrease in number, and the lightening of the color and texture may accomplish your goals. You may need touch-up treatments one to four times a year initially to maintain the improvement. About 10 percent of people are resistant to any type of hair-removal laser.

Quick Dos and Don'ts for Laser Hair Removal

- Don't pluck, wax, bleach, or have electrolysis for three to four weeks (for the face) or ten weeks (for the body) before your treatment.
- It's fine to shave the area up to the day before.
- Don't tan at all for four weeks.
- Don't use self-tanners for two weeks.
- Do tell your doctor about any medication changes.

"Do laser treatments hurt?"

There may be mild discomfort during treatment, which tends to be about the equivalent of a very light snap of a rubber band. But few people discontinue laser hair reduction due to discomfort; most people, in fact, tolerate it easily. Some dermatologists recommend purchasing a gentle numbing cream such as ELA-Max (lidocaine) that you can apply approximately 30 minutes before treatment. This may make the treatment more comfortable. Also, taking acetaminophen the night before and morning of the treatment may help with any discomfort you may have.

"How long do laser hair-removal treatments take?"

Treatments can take anywhere from several minutes to several hours or more depending on the size of treatment area and the type of laser being used. Small areas on the face might take 15 to 30 minutes; a bikini line may take 20 to 40 minutes depending on the laser system used and the amount of hair; and both full legs might take from 45 to 90 minutes. Some lasers have special heads or scanners that speed up the treatment. If time is a premium for you, be sure to ask about this before you tackle large areas such as the legs or back.

"What do I need to do before having laser hair reduction?"

You can maximize your results by doing (or not doing) the following:

1. It's very important that you don't tan. If you've had *any* sun exposure in the month prior to your laser hair-removal treatment, be sure to notify the nurse or doctor. Tanning of any type changes the laser settings and is the most common cause of complications after treatment. This also includes self-tanners—be sure that you don't use these for two weeks before any laser hair removal.

2. Don't pluck, wax, bleach, have electrolysis, or use depilatory creams for at least three to four weeks for the face and ten weeks for the body prior to the treatment. The hair must be present for the laser to find it.

3. Laser hair reduction works best when there's short stubble. You may be asked to shave the day before the treatment if the hair is long.

4. Take off any makeup or lotion prior to your treatment.

5. If you're taking antibiotics or any new medications, be sure to inform your nurse or dermatologist prior to the treatment. Medications can cause blistering and other complications, and your laser practitioner may need to change the settings of the laser to adjust for the medication.

6. If you're having your bikini line treated, wear light-colored panties in the shape you'd like your bikini line to be. The laser is absorbed by dark colors, and you want the hair to absorb the laser light, not your panties. Some offices have paper panties for you to wear.

7. Check with your doctor before taking aspirin, ibuprofen, or naproxen for the week prior to your laser treatment. Acetaminophen may be safely taken for pain or headaches.

"Can I continue to use my normal skin-care products while I'm receiving laser hair treatments?"

Many dermatologists will permit you to continue to use Renova cream, other vitamin-A derivatives, alpha-hydroxy acids, topical vitamin C, and any other products that you regularly use. But you should check with your dermatologist just to be sure.

"What should I expect during the laser treatment?"

At the first visit, you'll be asked to read and sign a consent form, and photos may be taken. You should also be given appropriate eye protection for safety reasons. If the laser wand doesn't have a cooling tip built into it, cooling gel may be applied to your skin. The laser practitioner will then pass the laser handpiece over the area you want treated.

The laser beam follows the hair shaft down into the follicle and heats it. The injured follicle will produce a weaker, finer hair—or no hair at all—on the next growth cycle. Some hairs will be thinned during the treatment, and some may be shed after one to seven days. Shaving is fine, but the remaining hairs should not be plucked or tweezed.

"What will my skin look like after the treatment?"

Your skin may have a slightly pink or sunburned look and may have tiny red bumps at the site of the hair follicles. This is temporary and is a good sign that the laser has heated the follicle. But don't worry if you don't see immediate redness: Changes also take place under the skin, and lasers can work without causing any redness, too.

"Are there specific instructions following the treatment?"

Be sure to carefully follow any and all instructions your dermatologist gives you. For instance, your skin should be handled very gently, and cool ice packs are usually fine if the area feels slightly warm. If your dermatologist okays it, one-percent hydrocortisone, Solarcaine gel, or aloe-vera gel may be applied. You may be asked to use a topical antibiotic ointment such as Polysporin if there's a break in the skin.

It's extremely important that you never pick, scratch, or scrub skin that's had recent laser treatments, as that could cause scarring. Ask your doctor if you should be using your normal skin-care products. Usually it's a good idea to take a break from products containing alpha-hydroxy acids or vitamin A for a week or so if the skin is irritated after your laser treatment. Again, dermatologists vary somewhat on this, so be sure to ask yours what she recommends.

"What problems should I report to my dermatologist after treatment?"

Be sure to call her if you have any breaks in the skin or blistering after a laser treatment—usually the skin will heal just fine, but your doctor should know about it. You may be asked to use special antibiotic ointment or dressings in this instance. While there's often a little bit of redness for a couple of days, if the redness increases or the area becomes hot, sore to the touch, or if there's any visible pus or yellow crusting, be sure to call your doctor right away, as these symptoms may indicate infection. Also, if you have a history of staph infections, it isn't a bad idea to let your dermatologist know that before starting treatment.

"I seem to be getting dark marks at spots where the laser is hitting. Is this normal?"

Many different types of laser treatments can produce these dark marks, particularly if you have a darker skin type, meaning skin that ranges from olive or dark golden (that tans easily and almost never burns) to the darkest African-American skin. If you do have a darker skin type, your dermatologist will automatically adjust the laser settings to try to avoid temporary darkening of the skin.

If some darkening (called *post-inflammatory hyperpigmentation*) occurs, it's almost always temporary and will usually go away in one to six months. Your dermatologist may ask you to take a break from your laser hair-treatment schedule in order to let the skin rest, or she may prescribe a "bleaching cream" to help it resolve faster.

If this darkening happens to you, be sure to protect yourself well every single day with a sunscreen containing zinc, as any unprotected light exposure will make the dark spots last longer and more difficult to treat. Also, invest in a good, wide-brimmed hat to wear on sunny days.

"What are the best laser hair-reduction and maintenance systems?"

There are three main laser hair-reduction systems and a number of other systems that are all safe and effective in experienced hands. The three main systems are the alexandrite laser, the diode laser, and the intense pulsed light system (a close laser cousin) sometimes known as the *EpiLight*—several different companies make each of these lasers under different trade names. Be sure to look for a laser clinic where either a dermatologist-supervised RN, a certified physician's assistant, or the doctor does the treatment.

There's always some debate about the relative advantages of one system over another. Many of the physician proponents of one particular laser system are paid to be consultants or researchers by that same laser company. In my opinion, that makes it difficult for the doctor in question to be completely objective about other laser systems. Physicians also tend to prefer systems that they're experienced on and comfortable with, which also creates a slight prejudice.

The intense pulsed light systems have a slight advantage for darker skin types because they have more flexibility with the exact wavelength used and other settings. However, experienced laser operators can get nice results with most laser systems.

Keep in mind that laser hair research is very active right now—new lasers are being tested and marketed all the time. But be extremely wary of the marketing hype surrounding laser systems. It's best to stick with systems that are tried and true until a new laser has at least a one- to two-year track record.

SUMMARY OF UNWANTED HAIR: WHAT TO DO

If you have a small amount of unwanted hair, traditional "physical" methods of plucking, waxing, and shaving work fine. The two disadvantages to these methods, as we all know, are that they're temporary (because they remove the hair at the surface of the skin) and can be uncomfortable. If you have a small amount of unwanted hair that's gray or blonde, try Vaniqa cream. For a more permanent solution to unwanted hair in limited places, try electrolysis.

To remove larger areas of unwanted hair more effectively, consider laser hair reduction. The cost of treatment varies so much by the site treated, the geographic area you live in, and the type of clinic you go to, that it's not possible for me to give you meaningful cost information here.

While laser hair reduction works well, it has some risks associated with it and is more expensive in the short term. But if you add up all the costs of the other methods you're using over a three- to five-year period, you might be surprised by how they compare with the laser. And laser hair reduction is the best, most effective solution to larger or stubborn areas of hair. It's given significant relief to many people who were painfully self-conscious about their unwanted hair.

๑๑ ๑๑ ๑๑   ๑๑ ๑๑ ๑๑

PART IV

SKIN HEALTH AND SUNSCREEN

12

PROMOTING SKIN HEALTH

It would be nice if there were a magic pill, lotion, or food that could instantly make skin perfect. But skin health, like your health in general, can't be improved by any one thing. Many factors, such as genetics, lifestyle, skin care, sun protection, diet, and illness reveal themselves—positively or negatively—in your skin.

I've already covered several of these topics earlier in the book, but in this chapter, I'd like to focus on promoting skin health through nutrition and diet, and also address some lifestyle issues. Your diet clearly affects the health and beauty of your skin, just as it does your general health. Positive eating habits and lifestyle choices can go a long way toward improving the appearance of dull, yellow, or ashy skin.

WHAT CAN IMPROVE YOUR SKIN?

- A healthy diet
- Weight control
- Vitamin and mineral supplements (and topical creams)

WHAT CAN AFFECT YOUR SKIN ADVERSELY?

- Smoking
- Chemotherapy
- Diabetes
- Medications

WHAT CAN IMPROVE YOUR SKIN?

A Healthy Diet

"For years I didn't pay much attention to what I ate, and now my skin just doesn't look good anymore. Are there any foods that can help my skin?"

It's easier to get away with poor eating habits when we're 18—that bag of potato chips won't show up in our faces (or our tushes) quite as much. That's less true as time goes by, as you've found out. We are what we eat, and this adage applies as much to skin as much as it does to any other organ in the body. However, it's never too late to improve on your nutritional habits, so the answer to your question is a definite *yes.*

If your daily diet is filled with an abundance of white sugar and flour, unhealthy fats and oils, sodas, coffee, and too much alcohol, then your skin isn't getting the nutrients it needs to be healthy. And skin *needs* to be healthy in order to be beautiful.

Occasional or very small amounts of the foods mentioned above aren't really the issue; problems arise when you eat those foods a lot. In addition, their empty calories will reduce your appetite for healthy foods. For example, if you begin breakfast with a large doughnut, chances are you won't want a bowl of whole-grain cereal or oatmeal with raisins right afterwards—you'll be too full! And a slice of pizza (laden with high-fat cheese, salt, and white flour) at 4:30 may be yummy, but your healthy dinner at 6:00 will probably suffer from that choice.

We need healthy food to have healthy skin, so keep your diet balanced with protein-rich foods such as fish, chicken, and other lean meats; lots of fresh vegetables and fruits; and complex carbohydrates such as whole-grain breads, cereals, and brown rice, or other grains.

The good news is that if you improve your diet and gradually eliminate junk food, your skin will look better—*much* better. Expect to see the changes occur slowly over a two- to twelve-month period. You'll be happy with the results, and the rest of your body will thank you, too.

"If I eat a lot of protein, especially fresh salmon and other fish, will I have nice skin?"

A number of patients have asked me recently if eating a lot of salmon will keep their skin wrinkle free. While fish is an excellent source of protein, and fish oils are an outstanding source of fatty acids, eating a lot of fish in and of itself is not going to make your wrinkles disappear.

However, eating fish three or four times a week is a wonderful idea, for it's high in protein and in the fatty acids that help lower cholesterol and triglycerides, called *omega-3 fatty acids.* Since much of our body is made of protein, including our muscles, skin, nails, and hair, it's important to eat enough protein to allow these tissues to repair themselves on a daily basis.

While there's some disagreement about how much protein is adequate, most nutritionists recommend between 40 and 75 grams of protein a day for an adult woman depending on her age and level of activity. If you're pregnant, you may need even more, particularly if you're carrying twins.

Excellent sources of protein include the following (each of which is considered one protein serving): dairy products—24 ounces of milk, ¾ cup lowfat cottage cheese, 1¾ cup of plain yogurt, or half a cup of grated cheese; eggs—two whole eggs plus two egg whites; meat and fish—three to four ounces of lean chicken, fish, shrimp, lean beef, lamb, or pork; or five ounces of crab or other shellfish.

Vegetarians, particularly vegans, should consume at least four protein servings a day. Protein sources could include tofu; legumes (many different types of beans); whole grains (such as brown rice, barley, or millet); soy pasta; whole-grain cereals; nuts and seeds; and dairy products (if those are eaten).

"I'm confused—which fats are good for you and which are not?"

This is a very hot topic right now. And while I can't give you every different viewpoint or scientific fact on fat, I can give you some practical suggestions for a healthy, balanced diet—including which fats should be avoided and which ones are okay.

Good fats. Certain fats, such as linoleic acid, are important for the formation of cell membranes, which are the outer linings of skin cells that allow the plasticity necessary in skin. Deficiencies of these essential fatty acids in animals have long been known to cause scaliness of the skin, problems in maturation of skin cells, and increased water loss throughout the skin. If these animals are then fed linoleic acids, the changes reverse and their skin becomes healthy again.

Other good fats are omega-3 polyunsaturated fatty acids or omega-3 fatty acids such as DHA (docosahexaenoic acid). DHA has been shown to help lower cholesterol and blood pressure as well as reduce the risk of heart disease. Research has also shown that it's essential for proper brain growth and eye development in a developing fetus.

So, where can you find healthy fatty acids such as DHA and linoleic acid? Good sources are oily fish such as salmon or trout; DHA-rich eggs (found in many supermarkets); and flaxseed, regular eggs, tuna, crab, and shrimp (which contain smaller amounts).

Extra virgin olive oil is not only great in salad dressings, but it's also one of the most health-promoting types of oils available. In America, high fat intake is associated with diseases such as heart disease, diabetes, and colon cancer. In many other parts of the world, however, a high fat intake actually is associated with lower rates of these conditions. It turns out that olive oil accounts for a high proportion of the fat intake in countries with low rates of these diseases, and it may also help lower cholesterol. But it's important to use olive oil *in place of* other fats—don't just add it to a diet already high in unhealthy fats.

"How much is too much?"

The average American, unfortunately, gets 40 percent (or even more) of their calories from fat. That's not good, especially when, according to current nutritional guidelines, no more than 30 percent of an adult's calories should come from fat—and many nutrition experts recommend even less, more in the range of 15 to 20 percent. This means that if you weigh 140 pounds and need approximately 2,200 to 2,500 calories a day to support a semi-active lifestyle, then no more than 600 to 700 of your daily calories should come from fat. (These guidelines may be changing to allow more "healthy" fats.)

Bad fats. All fats should be eaten in balance with other foods, but there are two types that you should seriously limit. You probably already know about saturated fats, which are fats that are solid at room temperature, such as butter. Saturated fats have a rigid molecular structure that tends to be incorporated into the cell that picks up these fat molecules, which is why saturated fats are associated with heart diseases such as hardening of the arteries.

But the really bad fat is one created by humans, called *partially hydrogenated fat,* or *trans fat.* A hydrogenated fat is made by bubbling hydrogen into an oil, such as palm, safflower, soy, or corn. These trans fats are difficult to metabolize, incorporate into cell structures, or excrete. So they simply remain stuck in our circulation, contributing significantly to the risk of heart disease and possibly cancer.

Trans fats are labeled on foods as various oils that are "partially hydrogenated," and they're everywhere. They appear in potato chips, cookies, crackers, and many other processed and baked foods. Most fast-food French fries are cooked in these partially hydrogenated oils . . . and Americans consume an average of 30 pounds of French fries a year.

How bad are these partially hydrogenated oils? A recent study of almost 80,000 women found that just a 5-percent increase in consumption of saturated fats increases the risk of heart disease by 17 percent—yet only a 2-percent increase in consumption of the trans fats in partially hydrogenated oils increases the risk of heart disease by 93 percent!

So the bottom line on fats is to eat oily fish, DHA-rich eggs, olive oil, and other vegetable oils in moderation. Eat butter, lard, and saturated fats in very limited amounts, and avoid baked or fried foods containing partially hydrogenated oils as much as you can.

"Will eating a high-fiber diet help my skin?"

A high-fiber diet by itself has never been proven to make skin look better. But because such a diet will most likely improve digestion and elimination and will help prevent constipation and possibly colon cancer, it's an excellent way to eat anyway. Since high-fiber foods are primarily fresh fruits, vegetables, and whole grains, these are foods that impart many nutritional benefits on their own. In fact, many nutritionists recommend four to six servings of fresh fruits, vegetables, and whole grains a day.

Weight Control

"Does how much I weigh affect my skin?"

Weight and good skin do not necessarily correlate. After all, there are many overweight women who have nice skin; conversely, there are many slender women whose skin isn't particularly good.

But being overweight does contribute to health problems, particularly heart disease, high blood pressure, diabetes, and joint problems. And large fluctuations in weight over the years may result in more wrinkles as the skin is repeatedly stretched and shrunk.

Weight loss is a very important topic. Some of us battle weight our entire lives, while others simply put on a few extra pounds as they age. And the causes of weight gain are not only controversial but also vary among different people: For some, genetics play a powerful role; for others, life experience and psychological issues are paramount.

Keep in mind that exercise boosts circulation to the skin, which can have a very positive effect on both your outer appearance and your inner self-image. Anything you can do to get moving for 15 to 20 minutes a day will really have a beneficial effect.

However, this isn't a book about weight control. There are plenty of excellent diet and nutrition books available now; and if you haven't already, you might visit **www.worldshealthiestfoods.com,** an excellent Website sponsored by the George Mateljan Foundation, a nonprofit foundation with no commercial interests or advertising.

Steps Toward Eating Better Now

1. Substitute olive oil for butter whenever you can.
2. Buy fresh fruit every time you go to the grocery store. If healthy snacks are available in your home, you'll be more likely to eat them instead of junk food.
3. Treat yourself to your favorite fish at least once a week.
4. Find some high-protein bars (such as Power Bars, Balance Bars, or Cliff Bars) that you like, and keep them everywhere: your car, gym bag, desk drawer, and so on. That way, you'll eat the bars when you're hungry instead of chips or sweets.
5. Splurge on your favorite nuts and cheeses so you have great high-protein snacks around (but keep in mind that a little of these foods goes a long way).

Vitamin and Mineral Supplements (and Topical Creams)

"Can vitamins improve the skin?"

This is an interesting and complicated question. There's quite a bit of data showing that certain vitamins, particularly C, E, and perhaps A, do act as antioxidants in the body. Antioxidants are thought to be beneficial because they help cells repair the damage done by aging and sunlight (along with other environmental insults).

It's difficult to document improvements in skin from vitamin tablets. But the research continues, and we don't know exactly what the final conclusion will be. In the meantime, it seems safe to say that small amounts of vitamins E, C, and A are probably not harmful and might very well be helpful. Taking pills with 200 to 800 extra units of vitamin E, 250 to 1,000 extra milligrams of vitamin C, and 5,000 extra units of vitamin A has no real downside, other than the expense, and may be beneficial. These amounts are present in most good multivitamins.

Be aware, however, that taking mega doses of any vitamin may be harmful. For example, taking vitamin A in excess can be toxic and can cause birth defects, among other things. Obstetricians recommend avoiding this vitamin (other than the amount in multivitamins) during pregnancy. This is also why doctors don't allow pregnant women to use Accutane (a drug for acne and a relative of vitamin A).

Antioxidants. Our cells are like little factories that produce energy. But unstable oxygen molecules, called *free radicals,* are a by-product of this energy production. The problem comes when free radicals damage parts of the cell by stealing electrons from other atoms in it. Antioxidants, often vitamins, snag those free radicals before they can do any damage to the cell.

The idea is that the more we can avoid habits that might generate extra free radicals, such as smoking or undue exposure to toxins, cigarettes, sunlight, and air pollution, the healthier we'll be over time. There's considerable debate about whether or not it's best to get these antioxidants from food or from supplements. Since healthy food has a lot of other benefits, it makes sense to me to get most of our antioxidants from food—however, I'm also a realist who knows that many of us don't ingest perfectly healthy diets and may not have access to fresh, organic fruits and vegetables. And so, if our diets are deficient, it makes sense to use supplements.

The most common antioxidants are discussed below.

Vitamin C. Vitamin C promotes tissue repair, including wound healing and many other metabolic processes; it also helps calcium absorption. Good sources of vitamin C include all citrus fruits and juices (particularly if they're fresh), mangoes, papayas, cantaloupe, strawberries, most berries, cooked broccoli, cauliflower, cabbage, and tomatoes. The general recommendation for vitamin C is 50 to 1,000 mg a day. There's a great deal of controversy about supplements, but if you eat two to four servings of vitamin-C-rich foods a day, you should be covered.

Vitamin A. This fat-soluble vitamin is known for protecting vision, but it also helps maintain the lining of the mouth, esophagus, and digestive tract. It supports healthy immune and reproductive systems and plays a vital role in bone development as well. Foods high in vitamin A include raw carrots, spinach, sweet potatoes, romaine lettuce, cantaloupe, fresh peppermint leaves, tomatoes, and bell peppers. Most nutritionists recommend approximately 5,000 units of vitamin A daily—don't take more because it can be stored in the fat in our bodies and cause toxicity.

Vitamin E. This vitamin helps protect your skin from ultraviolet light and prevents cell damage from free radicals. Vitamin E isn't a single substance but is actually a family of fat-soluble vitamins—some members of this family are called *tocopherols*. Good sources of vitamin E include spinach, sunflower seeds, broccoli, almonds, olives, papaya, and even bell peppers and blueberries. The current recommendations for this vitamin are very low: Most nutritionists recommend anywhere from 200 to 800 units a day depending on your age and health factors.

B vitamins. These are often referred to as *B complex* because there are many different vitamin Bs, including B_1, B_2, B_5, B_6, and B_{12}. The functions of B-complex vitamins are too numerous to go into here, but let's just say that they act as

helpers for the many hundreds of enzymes in the body that are necessary for healthy cellular function. These enzymes are particularly important for healthy nervous systems, hearts, and red blood cells.

Because you shouldn't take large amounts of one to the exclusion of others, B vitamins are usually sold as a complex or are already balanced in a multivitamin. If you're not sure if your multivitamin contains it, you can take a separate B-vitamin complex. (Also see **www.worldshealthiestfoods.com** for an in-depth discussion of each individual B vitamin.)

Minerals. Minerals are extremely important. The main ones that our body needs are calcium and magnesium, but trace minerals (such as selenium, zinc, copper, and chromium) are also important in small amounts. It's not a bad idea to take a multivitamin with these minerals to be sure that you get them, particularly if you eat a lot of processed foods

Be aware that most multivitamins don't contain enough calcium. Most women and men should be getting between 1,000 and 1,500 mg of calcium a day. Approximately 300 mg of calcium is contained in the following: eight ounces of milk; five ounces of calcium-fortified milk; a cup and a half of cottage cheese; an ounce and a half of regular cheese; a half cup of frozen yogurt; six ounces of calcium-fortified orange juice; 1¾ cups of broccoli (which is a lot of broccoli); and six ounces of calcium-fortified soy milk.

As for calcium supplements, they're a bit tricky since they come in three forms. The first type is naturally derived calcium from sources such as bone meal, oyster shell, and limestone. These are typically less expensive, but may also contain a significant amount of lead, which is a toxic chemical that can affect the brain, kidneys, and red blood cells. The second type, refined calcium carbonate, is also inexpensive, but isn't absorbed as well as some other forms of calcium. To improve absorption, take calcium carbonate with meals. The third and most easily absorbed calcium is calcium citrate, which is a little more expensive, but well worth the cost.

"Can creams or lotions with vitamins improve the skin?"

I'm often asked if topical creams and lotions are good for your skin, and if vitamins may be good for skin, aren't they even better taken together? The answer is that the right kinds of topical creams or lotions with the right kind of vitamins may help your skin.

Having said that, I want to caution you against expecting dramatic changes overnight. Vitamin creams, like most aspects of skin care, show that they're working over time, not instantly. There have been a lot of claims recently about the beneficial effects of "cosmeceuticals," which the FDA doesn't regulate the same way it does drugs. Therefore, these products' claims don't have to be proven—and so, products such as "instant face lifts" act primarily to instantly lift the money out of your pocket.

So which topical creams work? Tretinoin (a relative of vitamin A that's sold under the brand names Retin-A or Renova) has been shown in many excellent studies to improve skin in a number of ways; there's also a large body of scientific data that says that it boosts collagen production, decreases fine lines and wrinkles, improves brown spots and "age spots," and makes skin feel smoother. Tretinoin normalizes sun-damaged skin cells called *keratinocytes,* and boosts circulation by encouraging the formation of new blood vessels in the skin. Its downside is that it's only available by prescription and may cause irritation in some users (see below). In my opinion, tretinoin is still the gold standard for anti-aging creams, and newer products should strive to demonstrate in controlled studies that they're as good or better—unfortunately, such studies are rarely done.

If you're prescribed tretinoin, make sure to apply it only at night because light inactivates it—it will be completely useless in the daytime. Don't forget to use your sunscreen in the morning, as tretinoin will make you slightly more sun sensitive.

Alpha-hydroxy acids (including glycolic acid, lactic acid, malic acid, and a number of others) and topical vitamin C have considerable scientific data behind them to support their use as anti-aging products. Studies have also shown that both improve sun-damaged skin (as long as they're formulated correctly), with the effect being similar to that of tretinoin. Try alternating tretinoin with topical vitamin C or a glycolic acid preparation in the 10 to 15 percent range for extra benefit—they may also help remove any flaking that occurs as a side effect of tretinoin.

How to Reduce Irritation from Renova (Tretinoin)

If your skin gets irritated after using Renova, try the following measures, which may also work for topical vitamin-C or alpha-hydroxy acids.

1. Wash your face with a gentle cleanser and let it dry for 10 to 30 minutes.

2. After your face is dry, apply a pea-sized amount of Renova to cover the entire face (most people use too much).

3. Don't use other renewal products such as topical vitamin C or alpha-hydroxy products in the beginning.

4. Avoid facial scrubs until you're tolerating the Renova well.

5. Try using Renova every other or every third night if you're still having problems.

WHAT CAN AFFECT YOUR SKIN ADVERSELY?

Smoking

"I've smoked for ten years. My doctor told me that if I quit now, my skin will look better. Is this true?"

Yes. Smoking not only poisons the lungs, it also poisons the circulation in the skin. Smoking robs skin of the oxygen it needs, and the chemicals in cigarette smoke gradually destroy small blood vessels—which is why most smokers over the age of 30 have a very unhealthy grayish or yellowish tone to their skin. Also, since smokers are constantly pursing their lips to drag the smoke out of the cigarette, they develop very deep upper- and lower-lip lines as a result.

Quitting the smoking habit. The first step in your effort to stop smoking is to talk to your family doctor about programs that are available to help you. As with alcohol or drugs, quitting smoking can be difficult without a support group. There are just too many cues in daily life that trigger the desire for a cigarette. Most smokers have a number of these cues, such as finishing a meal, stress, lovemaking, camaraderie with co-workers, and so on. Since smoking is so interwoven into life habits, it can be very difficult to quit without help.

In addition to smoking-cessation programs, there are a number of medical aids that can help reduce the craving for nicotine during those first months when it's the strongest. Nicotine patches and gum can be extremely helpful when going through that withdrawal period.

There are also a number of excellent books available at any bookstore to inspire you to quit.

So, please talk to your doctor. Then ask your friends who have quit smoking for advice and see what they've found helpful for them. Your skin and entire body will thank you.

Chemotherapy

"I have breast cancer and am currently undergoing chemotherapy. My skin looks terrible—it's kind of a grayish color. Is this normal, and will it go away?"

Let me reassure you that this is completely normal. Many chemotherapy agents—whether they're being used for breast cancer, colon cancer, or any other type of cancer—work by killing rapidly dividing cells. This is a good treatment for cancer, because most tumors consist of mutated cells that are dividing more quickly than normal. But there are other noncancerous cells in the body that also divide rapidly, such as cells in the hair follicles, which chemotherapy also kills. This is why hair often falls out during treatment.

Skin, of course, doesn't fall off, but its normal cell-turnover rate decreases dramatically during chemotherapy. The top layer of healthy skin (known as the *epidermis*) normally completely renews itself every 30 to 45 days. During chemotherapy, however, the older dead layers of the skin aren't sloughing off as quickly as they used to, and the new, fresh skin cells aren't pushing up toward the epidermis as quickly. Consequently, the skin

often takes on a dullish gray or yellowish hue.

The good news is that this is temporary. As soon as your chemotherapy treatment ends, the skin cells will begin to turn over more rapidly. And the skin will usually return to normal within two to six months of stopping treatment.

Following are some things you can do during chemotherapy to help yourself feel and look your best. (**Note:** Please discuss these recommendations with your doctor to make sure that they agree with them.)

1. If you're still smoking, stop. I'm sure your doctor has already told you that.

2. Eat a balanced diet that's rich in protein, because skin cells are mostly made up of protein. Fish, chicken, and lean meats are excellent. Also, make sure that you eat several servings of vegetables and fruit each day. Try not to eat processed carbohydrates such as potato chips and other junk food. Brown rice, whole-grain breads, and potatoes with the skin on them are excellent substitutes. Cakes, cookies, and other foods containing refined sugars should really play a limited role in your diet, as your body needs to make every mouthful count right now.

3. Think about your diet the way you would if you were pregnant. You'd want to give your unborn child the very best nutrition possible, which is exactly what your body needs during chemotherapy.

4. Anything that improves the circulation is excellent for your skin: Exercise, steam rooms, hot tubs, and saunas in moderation may help your skin look healthier. Again, check with your doctor, because it's possible that an excess of heat might lower your blood pressure too much or be otherwise harmful.

5. Try massage therapy, which feels great and will temporarily help improve your circulation.

Diabetes

"I've had diabetes for 15 years, and my skin seems to look worse each year. Is there anything I can do to reverse this?"

To my knowledge, there haven't been any studies done to specifically look at diabetes and treatments that would improve the appearance of the skin. But most diabetics know that skin care is crucial to combat infections that can attack them through their skin. Let's cover some basics and then discuss the appearance of the skin, particularly the face.

Over time, diabetes usually causes poor circulation by narrowing small blood vessels all over the body, especially in the hands, lower legs, and feet. Many people already have poor circulation in their extremities anyway, so when you add the effect of diabetes, feet can become a real problem area. And the problem tends to be infection—poor circulation essentially reduces the body's ability to fight it off, which is why it's so important to maintain very good hygiene in the foot and nail area.

If you have diabetes, you probably already know that it's crucial that your feet don't get infected. You may not know, however, that infections of the feet can develop through tiny cracks in the skin, which are sometimes so small that you can't even see them. These microscopic cracks are often caused by common garden-variety athlete's foot (which is a fungus). So make sure that you use an anti-fungal cream on your feet regularly, or if you have athlete's foot, get it treated promptly. And if you have fungus in your toenails, it's important to get that treated as well. See your dermatologist.

Circulation to the face is affected slightly by diabetes, but not as much as the extremities. Problems with infections on the face aren't common unless the disease is quite advanced. Nevertheless, if you have diabetes, it's even more important to adopt all the healthy habits you can. This includes exercise, nutritious eating, not smoking, and keeping your blood sugar in check.

You may want to try microdermabrasion or facials, as you could enjoy the temporary boost in circulation. If nothing else, a facial can help you relax and de-stress for an hour, which is never harmful!

Medications

"I have rheumatoid arthritis and have to take a lot of different medications. Could they be making my skin look worse?"

It's possible, but it may just be that your overall health isn't good right now. Some medications used to treat diseases such as rheumatoid arthritis *can* have an effect on the cell-turnover rate. If taken for a long time, prednisone in particular will thin the skin, cause blood vessels to dilate, and make it difficult for the skin to heal. Long-term prednisone use also increases the growth of fine, usually blonde hairs all over the face (called *vellus hairs*) and causes fluid retention that can make the skin look puffy.

Some of the newer anti-inflammatory medications for arthritis have fewer side effects that affect the skin. Please discuss them with your rheumatologist or primary-care physician to see if they might be appropriate for you.

๑๑ ๑๑ ๑๑

In order to have the healthiest possible skin, people of all ages can benefit from eating more healthfully, exercising, using skin-renewal products, and having microdermabrasion or facials done. Over time, that improved circulation may reduce an ashy or yellowish tone, and restore the skin to a healthier color. If you have a particular problem or your skin doesn't seem to be responding to this chapter's suggestions, ask your dermatologist what she recommends.

๑๑ ๑๑ ๑๑   ๑๑ ๑๑ ๑๑

13

EVERYTHING YOU NEED TO KNOW ABOUT SUNSCREEN

I know that a lot of people grew up lusting after deep bronze tans. But as many baby boomers are finding out, that beautiful tan at age 20 will turn skin into what looks and feel like blotchy leather at 50. And *tanning booths are no better than the sun.* In fact, in some ways they're worse—as you read further in this chapter, you'll find out why I call tanning booths "wrinkle salons."

Someday, we may all be a rich mocha color, with no threat of skin cancer whatsoever. Or perhaps the fashion weather vane will swing around and start to prize the skin color that we were born with. My guess is that as the vast numbers of female baby boomers begin to see the damage inflicted by the sun firsthand, they'll start to value natural skin color in themselves and their children again. But in the meantime, you need to protect yourself from the sun. This chapter will give you the scoop on sunscreen.

WHAT YOU NEED TO KNOW

- Sunscreening 101
- The SPF rating system
- Choosing a sunscreen
- Children and sun protection
- UVA, UVB, and tanning
- Sunburn and its effects

WHAT YOU NEED TO KNOW

Sunscreening 101

"Who needs to use sunscreen?"

To make a long story short, nearly everyone! Even the darkest skin can burn, although it may not happen until you've spent a lot of time in the tropics or the mountains.

The Food and Drug Administration (FDA) and the American Academy of Dermatology (AAD) recognize six skin types (see below). If you have a skin type of I–III, it's recommended that you use sunscreen with an SPF of at least 15 every day regardless of the weather—particularly if you or your family have a history of sun damage, precancerous lesions, or skin cancer.

What Skin Type Am I?

1. Do you always burn easily and never tan, and are you extremely sun-sensitive? Are you a Caucasian of Irish, Scottish, or Welsh descent; or do you have red hair and freckles? If this describes you, then you're **Type I.**

2. Do you always burn easily, tan minimally, and have very sun-sensitive skin? Are you a Caucasian with fair skin and hair and blue eyes? If this describes you, then you're **Type II.**

3. Do you sometimes burn, tan gradually to a light brown, yet have sun-sensitive skin? Are you a dark-haired Caucasian or Asian with average skin? If this describes you, then you're **Type III.**

4. Do you burn minimally, always tan to a moderate brown, and have minimally sun-sensitive skin? Are you a Caucasian of Mediterranean descent; or a light-skinned African American, Asian, Hispanic, Indian, or Middle Eastern person? If this describes you, then you're **Type IV.**

5. Do you rarely burn, tan well, and have sun-insensitive skin? Are you Middle Eastern, Asian, Hispanic, Indian, or African American? If this describes you, then you're **Type V.**

6. Does your skin never burn, and are you sun-insensitive? Are you a deeply pigmented African American? If this describes you, then you're **Type VI.**

"How much sunscreen should be used, and how often should it be put on?"

You should apply sunscreen to dry skin 30 minutes before going outdoors. Pay special attention to your face, hands, arms, and shoulders (if they're exposed). One ounce, about enough to fill a shot glass, is needed to properly cover such areas of the body. Don't forget your ears if you have short hair. And lips can get sunburned, too—so be sure to apply a lip balm containing a sunscreen with an SPF of 15 or higher.

Sunscreen should be applied in the morning and reapplied after swimming or perspiring heavily. So-called water-resistant sunscreens lose their effectiveness after approximately 60 to 90 minutes in the water; and sunscreens rub as well as wash off, so if you dry off with a towel, reapply for continued protection. Keep in mind that you're exposed to the sun whenever you're outside, even on cloudy days.

"When should sunscreen be used?"

Every day—especially if you're in a high-risk group for skin cancers or want to prevent wrinkles. Most of us underestimate how much reflection we get from the sun: 17 percent of its rays are reflected back to us when we're on the sand, and 80 percent are reflected by the snow. Also, 40 to 80 percent of the sun's ultraviolet rays pass through clouds.

Don't forget that sun protection is the principal means of preventing premature aging and skin cancers: When used on a regular basis, sunscreen allows the skin to repair itself somewhat from previous damage. Sunscreen can be applied under makeup, and many cosmetic products today even come with an added SPF for daily use.

Because sun exposure is responsible for vitamin-D production in the skin, many adults who use sunscreen regularly may require supplements. Take a multivitamin daily, or drink your milk—vitamin-D supplements are often found in dairy products. Even many calcium supplements contain vitamin D.

The SPF Rating System

"What does SPF stand for?"

SPF stands for *sun protection factor*. It's calculated by comparing the amount of time needed to produce a sunburn on protected skin to the amount of time needed to cause a sunburn on unprotected skin.

Take, for example, a fair-skinned person who would normally turn red after ten minutes in the sun. If a sunscreen prolongs that 10 minutes to 50, then it earns an SPF of 5. A sunscreen with an SPF of 20 allows that person to multiply their initial burning time by 20. Our hypothetical fair-skinned person could then be in the sun for 200 minutes before turning red.

The misleading element of the SPF rating system is that it measures only the burn time, or UVB rays. It doesn't help at all in protecting skin from UVA radiation. These rays, as research has shown in the past few years, causes just as much risk as UVB for skin cancers, premature skin aging, and wrinkles—they just don't cause as much burning.

"Does SPF 30 have twice as much sun protection as SPF 15?"

No. SPF protection *does not* increase proportionately with the number. An SPF of 30 blocks 97 percent of the sun's burning rays (technically, the sunscreen absorbs or reflects the harmful radiation rather than letting it into the skin); an SPF of 15 absorbs 93 percent of the burning rays; and an SPF of 2 absorbs 50 percent of the sun's burning rays. If you're confused, you're not alone. Unfortunately, SPF ratings aren't particularly logical, and it would certainly have been easier if the SPF system had been developed so that a 30 was twice as effective as a 15. (Also remember that SPF tells you nothing about harmful UVA rays.)

Yet, in spite of the confusion, the SPF system will give you a rough measure of UVB protection. Recent research indicates that high-SPF sunscreens are still appropriate for very sun-sensitive skin types I and II. One study showed that an SPF of 15 produced two and a half times the number of sunburned cells as was seen with a SPF 30 with the same dose of sunlight. More research is under way, but the bottom line is, if you're very sun sensitive, use an SPF of 30 or above. And apply lots of it—as I've repeatedly said, most people tend to apply too little sunscreen.

"Does the SPF system tell how well a sunscreen blocks UVA and UVB rays?"

No. The SPF number on sunscreens only refers to how well the product protects from UVB rays. At present, there's no FDA-approved rating system that identifies UVA protection. It helps to look for sunscreens that say "broad spectrum" on them, but even this isn't very accurate.

Scientists are working on a way to create a standardized testing system to measure UVA protection, but in the meantime, think zinc! Sunscreens containing 4 to 7 percent zinc are best at blocking UVA rays. Parsol 1789/avobenzone is also an excellent UVA blocker. Titanium is good, too, but it's my third choice.

Choosing a Sunscreen

"How do I choose the right sunscreen?"

There are so many different types of sunscreens that selecting the right one can be very confusing.

For the best protection, use a sunscreen containing zinc or Parsol 1789/avobenzone to block UVA radiation. Use an SPF of 15 or higher—if you're very sun sensitive, use an SPF of 30 or more.

As for the form of the sunscreen, gels are best for acne-prone skin, while lotions and creams are fine provided that you apply enough and they don't cause breakouts. Look for one that says *noncomedogenic* (which means it won't make your acne worse). If you still feel unsure, your dermatologist should be able to recommend one that doesn't aggravate your acne.

All sunscreens need to be reapplied. Those that are water resistant should be reapplied about every two to three hours, immediately after swimming, or during activities where you might be sweating a lot. Gels, lotions, and creams that aren't water-resistant need to be reapplied very frequently, as they wear off easily.

Most sunscreens these days don't contain PABA (or *para-aminobenzoicacid*) because it stains clothes and causes fairly frequent allergic reactions. You should definitely avoid it.

Which Sunscreen Should I Buy?

I recommend that you purchase three different kinds of sunscreen: one for daily use for your face, neck, chest, and hands; one for the same areas for outdoor sports, vacations, and other high-sun activities; and one for your body. I understand that the many shelves of sunscreen in the drugstore can be fairly daunting, so here are some suggestions:

1. **Daily use**. Every morning, you should apply this product right after you've washed your face. It should go under anything else, such as foundation or moisturizer. It must block both UVA and UVB to be really effective, so it should contain zinc, Parsol 1789, or titanium. Try Cetaphil Facial Moisturizer SPF 15 (sold in drugstores), SkinCeuticals Sun Defense SPF 20 or 30 (found in dermatologists' offices), Clinique City Block SPF 15 (sold in department stores), Olay Complete UV-Protective Moisture Lotion (sold in drugstores), or M.D. Forté Environmental Protection Cream SPF 30 (found in dermatologists' offices).

2. **Outdoor sports and activities.** Next, for your face, neck, and chest especially, pick a product to be used in high-sun situations, such as vacations, swimming, and other outdoor sports and activities. Invest in a really good one that has at least 4 to 7 percent zinc, is waterproof, sweatproof, and has an SPF 30 or above. Try SkinCeuticals Sport SPF 45. (Keep in mind that these products tend to be rather expensive.)

3. **Your body.** Third, pick one for your body for times when you're outside swimming, working, or exercising but don't want to put the really expensive sunscreen all over your body. Try waterproof Coppertone Sport SPF 45 in the large bottles (sold in discount stores such as Costco).

"What's the difference between sunscreen and sunblock?"

Sunscreen chemically absorbs ultraviolet (UV) rays, while sunblock physically deflects them. New preparations for sunblock (such as micronized zinc or titanium dioxide) offer substantial UVA and UVB protection. These newer sunblocks pulverize the zinc into tiny particles (hence, the word *micronized*) so that they absorb into the skin well and aren't visible the way the older zinc preparations were. Regular zinc is great and is still available at stores that cater to rock climbers, mountaineers (try Recreational Equipment, Inc.: **www.rei.com**), and surfers. It even comes in fun colors such as blue or green.

"Is wearing sunscreen all I need to do to protect myself from the sun?"

No, particularly if you have a personal history of skin cancer or precancerous lesions or have a family history of melanomas or other skin cancers. Current sunscreens aren't completely protective—they'll allow some UV radiation in, no matter how good they are and how much you apply. Sunscreen should be viewed as a backup to the primary means of sun protection—such as wide-brimmed hats, protective clothing, and avoiding the sun between the peak hours of 10:00 A.M. and 3:00 P.M.

Children and Sun Protection

"Is it true that repeated sunburns in childhood increase the risk of skin cancer?"

A number of studies have shown that repeated sunburns do greatly increase the risk for melanomas (the type of skin cancers that can sometimes be fatal if not caught early).

It's extremely important to prevent sunburns in children, as they have many more years on this planet and more potential for repeated sun damage—all of which increases the risk for such cancers as melanoma. Also, some scientists think that the thinning of the ozone layer may have a major effect on our children and greatly increase their risks of skin cancer.

The Australians have developed very sleek and stylish sun-protective bathing suits for children. I like to call them "surfer suits." They have long sleeves, cover the legs to mid-calf, and look like extremely lightweight wetsuits. Most children like them—if they start wearing them when they're young, and their parents treat the suits as they would car seats (that is, nonnegotiable safety measures). The suits leave the face, neck, hands, and feet exposed, so they'll still need sunscreen. Visit **www.solumbra.com** to order one of these suits.

UVA, UVB, and Tanning

"What's the difference between UVA and UVB wavelengths?"

Sunlight consists of two types of harmful rays—UVB (290 nm–320 nm) and UVA (320 nm–400 nm).

UVB rays are the sun's "burning" rays and are the primary cause of sunburn and skin cancer. UVA rays, however, pass through window glass and car windows and penetrate deeper into the structural layer of the skin, called the *dermis*. This layer contains the elastic and collagen fibers that support the skin and give it tone and elasticity. UVA rays contribute to skin cancer, premature wrinkling, and sun damage, and to skin burning as well. In addition, both kinds of rays can cause suppression of the immune system in the skin, which protects one from the development and spread of skin cancer.

"Is there a safe way to tan?"

No. The only known safe way to tan is with self-tanners (creams or lotions you can put on the skin that give it a slightly golden glow without any of the injury of sun exposure).

Tanning occurs when the sun's ultraviolet rays penetrate the skin's outer layer, which causes the skin to produce more melanin (the brown color in skin) as a response to an injury. In spite of the claims that tanning booths offer safe tanning, these booths can actually cause sunburns, skin cancer, and premature aging of the skin. In other words, artificial radiation from tanning booths carries all the same risks of natural sunlight—including damaging the skin's immune system.

Many tanning salons are unregulated and allow customers to use their beds without supervision or eye protection. The American Academy of Dermatology supports local and statewide tanning-parlor regulations, and believes that warning signs should be prominently displayed in tanning salons listing the risks of tanning exposure.

Self-tanning creams, however, are safe. The top or outermost layer of skin is called *the stratum corneum*. It's made of dead skin cells, and there are no blood vessels there. Self-tanners just stain this outer dead layer a brown color, thus causing no harm to the skin.

Sunburn and Its Effects

"How should I treat a sunburn?"

First-degree burns are red and will usually heal (after some peeling) within a few days. The pain can be treated with cool baths—try Aveeno oatmeal bath as an additive to help soothe the skin. Nonirritating moisturizers such as Cetaphil lotion or over-the-counter hydrocortisone one-percent cream may make you more comfortable. Aspirin or ibuprofen taken early in the development of a sunburn may help prevent its extension, as a result of these medications' anti-inflammatory properties. It's best to avoid the use of benzocaine products, which can cause allergic reactions.

Second-degree sunburns blister and can be considered a medical emergency if a large area is affected. If a sunburn is severe, it may be accompanied by headaches, chills, or fever, and medical attention should be sought right away. Be sure to protect your skin from the sun while it heals, for you want to avoid the repeated burns that are associated with a greater risk for skin cancer.

☙☙ ☙☙ ☙☙   ☙☙ ☙☙ ☙☙

PART V

---◇---

COMMON SKIN PROBLEMS

14

HOW TO
HANDLE ACNE

For a substantial number of us, acne can be a torment. It afflicted us as teens, it plagues our own kids now, and it can linger even after menopause. Acne is a complicated topic because it exists in many forms and has many treatments. This chapter will help clear up some of the confusion and provide you with the information you need to ask your dermatologist the right questions.

WHAT YOU NEED TO KNOW

- What causes acne?
- The different grades of acne
- Acne and age

WHAT ARE THE POSSIBLE TREATMENTS?

- Topical medications
- Oral medications
- Microdermabrasion
- Facials

WHAT YOU NEED TO KNOW

What Causes Acne?

"No one else in my family seems to have acne, so why do I?"

Acne (or a history of it) does tend to run in families, but this is not always the case. While doctors understand the process of acne

167

pretty well, we just don't understand all of its causes or why it occurs in particular family members and not others. In any case, hormones are almost always to blame.

Both males and females experience surging hormones around ages 10 to 14 that stimulate the oil glands on the face, chest, and back to secrete more oil. These oil glands connect to hair follicles—which are like tiny canals for hair—and the oil empties onto the skin through the follicle. The overabundant oil (called *sebum*) gets mixed with dead skin cells from the hair follicle and forms a plug. As bacteria begin to grow in the mixture of oil and cells, chemicals are released that cause inflammation, breaking down the follicle. The oil, dead cells, and bacteria then spill into the surrounding skin, causing more inflammation, swelling, and pus.

How bad the acne is depends on how big the plug (called a *comedone*) is, how deep it is in the skin, and how much inflammation it causes. If the plug is close to the surface and there isn't much inflammation, you might just have a blackhead or whitehead. If it forms deeper down in the follicle, then you might have a red bump or a pustule. If it forms very deep down and there's a lot of inflammation in the area, then a cyst forms. It's this type of cystic acne that usually causes scarring.

The Different Grades of Acne

"There are five children in my family, and we all have acne. Our dermatologist has prescribed different treatments for all of us. Can you explain why?"

Yes. You all probably have different types of acne (which dermatologists have categorized in a numerical system from I to IV), and each type requires its own individual treatment.

Some of the material that follows may seem technical, but since this topic is so complicated, the best way for you to educate yourself is to roll up your sleeves and learn as much as you can.

Blackheads and whiteheads (grade I). Almost everyone has some of this in their teenage years, which is also called *comedonal acne,*. These blackheads and whiteheads are usually found in the T-zone area but can occur anywhere, and, depending how severe the acne is, there may be anywhere from a few to several hundred lesions. Grade-I acne can usually be treated with acne washes and topical treatments such as gels, lotions, or creams.

Red bumps (grade II). This type has comedones (blackheads and whiteheads) and red bumps (papules) and is usually more inflamed than the previous two types. Grade-II acne can be found all over the face, and is generally treated with acne washes, gels, lotions or creams, and sometimes with oral antibiotics.

Pustules (grade III). This type of acne surfaces when the red bumps from grade II contain pus. Sometimes these pustules can be very inflamed and lead to scarring. If you have just a few comedones and pustules, your doctor might prescribe acne washes and a gel, lotion, or cream. However, if the acne is more severe, she might recommend oral antibiotics, oral contraceptives, or in cases with scarring, Accutane.

Cystic acne (grade IV). This type of acne contains characteristics of the previous three grades, plus cysts that are tender, deep, and hard. If these cysts are causing permanent scarring, Accutane will probably be prescribed, as it's the most effective medication for this type of acne. If the cysts aren't so severe or there isn't any scarring, a combination of all of the above-mentioned treatments might be used (with the exception of Accutane).

Acne and Age

"I'm in my 40s now, but I've had acne since I was a teenager. It seems as if it's different now, but I still have it. Am I ever going to grow out of having acne?"

For many people, acne lasts throughout their entire reproductive lives. It tends to begin when hormones start to activate in early puberty, and it can last until menopause. However, with postmenopausal hormone replacement, some women have acne into their 50s, 60s, or even 70s depending on the type of hormone replacement used. Acne definitely changes over the decades, though: Teenage acne is quite different from postmenopausal acne and should be treated as such. Below is a summary.

Teenage acne. Most people starting their sexual development have at least mild acne at some point during their adolescence. Oil secretion definitely increases, and blackheads and whiteheads often develop. As the teen years progress (especially if there's a family history of severe acne), it can become quite severe, with large cysts and subsequent scarring.

Acne during these years tends to be unpredictable, because the hormone levels of teenagers fluctuate so much. Young women in particular have irregular cycles and menstrual periods that aren't established yet, so their estrogen and progesterone levels may be changing quite a bit from month to month. This is why your 16-year-old daughter's mild acne can turn severe in a matter of months.

In addition, most teenage acne is concentrated through what's called the T-zone (the forehead, nose, and chin), although it may go on to involve the cheeks; and young skin tends to be much oilier than older skin. But this is very individual: Some people have extremely oily skin that persists even into their 30s and 40s and tends to be acne prone even then; others have oily skin only in their teens, and by their 30s have drier, clearer skin.

Acne in the 20s and 30s. In most cases, skin at this stage is already beginning to be less oily and breakout prone than in the teens. Sometimes, though, acne may start in the 20s or 30s—even if the person had clear skin in their teenage years. Again, hormones are usually the culprits. Remember, if you've recently gone off oral contraceptives, this probably accounts for your more severe breakouts.

If your acne is mild, give non-prescription medications a try for two or three months, then see your dermatologist. However, if your acne is moderate to severe, make an appointment right away, but use the nonprescription medications until you can be seen by your dermatologist.

Acne breakouts in the 40s (perimenopausal acne). For most men, acne is gone by the time they reach their 40s—but this isn't necessarily the case for women. For some women, their 40s mean complete freedom from acne; for others, acne may actually worsen during the five to ten years prior to menopause (also known as *perimenopause*).

Menopause occurs in most women in their early 50s. But during perimenopause, our hormonal systems are already beginning to change, even though we're still having regular periods. Women in their 40s tend to notice that their periods are gradually getting lighter and may even notice late periods, which may indicate that ovulation didn't occur that month (called an *anovulatory cycle*).

Acne in the 40s is generally different from adolescent acne in that there aren't as many blackheads, whiteheads, papules, or pustules. Instead, it's more microcystic—that is, small, hard, tender cysts often occur around the chin, jawline, and sometimes down on to the neck. Severe acne with very large cysts (or *nodulocystic acne*) is rare in either

sex in the 40s, but the small cysts of microcystic acne are still capable of scarring if they get inflamed enough.

Postmenopausal acne. It used to be that women were entirely free of acne after menopause, but hormone replacement therapy (HRT) has changed all that.

HRT uses different types of estrogens, progesterones, and sometimes even testosterone to keep a postmenopausal woman's hormone levels appropriately balanced. The low-dose estrogen itself usually isn't a problem for the skin—more often it's the progesterone- or testosterone-related side of HRT that causes acne.

But HRT is complicated and individualized for each woman, and you're probably aware of the debate over whether HRT should be used at all. If you're undergoing this therapy, you may want to ask your dermatologist or gynecologist if switching to a different type of progesterone compound or a lower estrogen dose might be helpful to your skin. Many different types of progesterone exist, and you may find one that works for you without causing you to break out.

There's also a new IUD available that delivers progesterone right to the uterus where it's needed, without much systemic absorption. Usually acne isn't a problem if one of these are used, but you should know that insurance companies generally won't cover them for acne and that they can cost between $500 and $700.

ꙩꙩ ꙩꙩ ꙩꙩ

POSSIBLE TREATMENTS

"There are so many different types of treatment for acne now. Which one should I be using?"

Most acne can now be controlled, but there are so many options for treatment that you need a customized treatment plan. This is why having a good doctor is important.

If your acne is mild, it's perfectly fine to try over-the-counter remedies, most of which have benzoyl peroxide or alpha- or beta-hydroxy acids in them. If your acne is moderate or severe, make an appointment with your doctor. A good primary-care physician will be comfortable treating mild to moderate acne, but a dermatologist should treat severe acne.

In my opinion, one of the main goals of acne treatment is to prevent permanent scarring. If you're starting to scar, your dermatologist may quickly move to oral antibiotics, oral contraceptives, or Accutane. For less severe types of acne, cleansers, gels, lotions, and creams may be very effective, either used alone or in combination with oral medications.

Remember that discoloration is different from permanent scarring. Permanent scarring is a depressed, raised, or white area that doesn't go away. Discoloration is red or brown, the skin is soft and flat, there's no indentation or change in texture, and while it may last for months, it's almost always temporary.

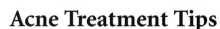

Acne Treatment Tips

1. Be patient. It takes eight to ten weeks to see if a new acne medication is working.
2. Apply creams, gels, or lotions in a thin layer over the entire area, not just on the lesions.
3. Don't pick! Picking can cause scars.
4. Stop the medicine and call your doctor if your skin is red or irritated for more than a couple of days.
5. Schedule a follow-up appointment in eight to ten weeks with your dermatologist.

Topical Medications

Washes. Most acne washes are formulated for oily skin and are appropriate for patients in their teens and 20s. Nonprescription washes usually contain benzoyl peroxide (either 5 or 10 percent) or glycolic or salicylic acids, but if your skin is dry or sensitive, these ingredients will probably just irritate you and should be avoided. Prescription washes, on the other hand, are usually a bit stronger, but they can be formulated to be less drying.

Acne medications can be irritating by themselves, so it may be best to use a gentle, nonirritating wash such as Cetaphil Gentle Skin Cleanser.

Gels, lotions, and creams. While nonprescription products are fine if you have very mild acne, you may need prescription items to make any real headway. Most over-the-counter gels, lotions, and creams (topical agents) contain low-strength benzoyl peroxide, a little alpha-hydroxy acid, salicylic acid, or retinol (which is *not* the same thing as Retin-A).

Fortunately, there are a lot of different prescription gels, lotions, and creams for your dermatologist to choose from now. Almost everyone can find something that will work for them, but you may need to try several until your doctor finds the right ones for your skin. Don't get discouraged if the results aren't instant: It takes eight to ten weeks to tell if an acne medicine is working.

Gels tend to be used for oily skin, whereas lotions and creams are usually prescribed for patients with dry or sensitive skin. Some of the choices include vitamin-A derivatives such as tretinoin (see below); Differin cream or gel, which is related to vitamin A but may be slightly less irritating; and Tazorac, which can be irritating.

Tretinoin. Sold under the brand names of Renova, Retin-A, Avita, or Retin-A Micro, this class of vitamin-A relatives works well for most types of acne. A secondary benefit is that tretinoin has been clearly shown to help reduce wrinkling over time. Renova is even formulated in a moisturizing base to facilitate use in older, drier skin. The concentration of tretinoin probably doesn't matter very much, as excellent effects over time are seen with lower concentrations—higher concentrations definitely cause more irritation but don't necessarily work better.

Unfortunately, tretinoin causes irritation in many people, but before you give up on it, make sure you're using it correctly. To do so, you need to do the following:

1. Wash your face with a very gentle cleanser and dry it thoroughly.

2. Wait 10 to 30 minutes before applying the cream to reduce the chance of skin irritation.

3. Spread one pea-sized amount gently over the *entire* face—don't just dot it on lesions.

4. Apply tretinoin at night because sunlight makes it inactive.

5. Be sure to use a sunscreen with an SPF of 15 or greater in the morning since the vitamin-A derivative may make you slightly more sensitive to the sun.

6. Avoid waxing, scrubs, or depilatories that may irritate the skin, and if you're having a facial or microdermabrasion, be sure to let your aesthetician know

ahead of time that you're using tretinoin.

Azelex. This is a relatively new but excellent treatment for mild to moderate acne. It's usually used twice a day and is significantly less irritating than vitamin-A derivatives. Some doctors recommend it in combination with other topical agents, so that Retin-A, for example, would be used at night and Azelex in the morning.

Benzamycin gel. This combination of benzoyl peroxide and erythromycin (a topical antibiotic) is excellent for mild to moderate acne, and is less irritating than vitamin-A derivatives but slightly more irritating than Azelex. Its one disadvantage is that it has to be stored in the refrigerator. However, it does last for about a week out of the refrigerator, so you can put a week's supply in your bathroom and then refill it weekly from the refrigerated container.

Topical antibiotics. There are a number of antibiotics that come in gel, lotion, or cream form. Some of the most common are clindamycin, erythromycin, and metronidazole (usually used for rosacea). These are often prescribed for mild to moderate acne and may be used alone but are more often used in conjunction with one of the above-mentioned topical medications.

Oral Medications

"My dermatologist prescribed minocycline for me, but I really don't like to take antibiotics on a regular basis. Why can't I just use a cream?"

Moderate to severe acne typically doesn't get better just with topical medications because the inflammation is too advanced and the plug in the hair follicle is too deep. A more systemic medication such as an antibiotic can usually tackle the deeper inflammation and bacterial growth in the follicle.

Oral antibiotics fight the bacteria in the lesion and some have anti-inflammatory properties as well. Some of the most commonly prescribed include minocycline, doxycycline, tetracycline, or erythromycin (or amoxicillin or penicillin derivatives if you're allergic to the others). Oral antibiotics are usually taken once or twice a day—some need to be taken on an empty stomach, so be sure to check with your doctor or pharmacist.

One strategy is to start with various washes, gels, or creams and use them for two or three months. If at the end of two or three months there hasn't been much response, your dermatologist might then add an oral antibiotic to take for several months or even up to several years. Another strategy is to start acne washes, gels, or creams at the same time with an oral antibiotic; if you're doing well by your next checkup, your dermatologist might then discontinue or taper off the oral antibiotic.

The trend in dermatology is to prescribe oral antibiotics less frequently and for more limited time periods because we've realized that using them for acne over long periods of time helps to breed antibiotic resistance in our society as a whole and in individuals as well. In addition, many women are prone to vaginal yeast infections while they're taking antibiotics. And other treatments have lessened our reliance on antibiotics; having said that, there are still some situations where they really are the best choice for treating acne. This is why it is important to have your treatment individualized by a dermatologist.

Oral contraceptives. Oral contraceptives can be very effective in treating acne, particularly for women in their late teens, 20s, and 30s, because they stabilize hormone levels from month to month. But it's wise to keep in mind that if you go off the Pill, your acne will almost certainly get worse, perhaps not right away, but within several months.

The first medication to be approved by the FDA for use in both birth control and the treatment of acne was Ortho Tri-Cyclen, but there are now several others that have been approved (or are in the process of being approved) for this use as well. Oral contraceptives can be used in combination with topical medications. Be aware that there have been a few reports that taking antibiotics may decrease the effectiveness of the Pill, so it may help to take these medications at different times of day.

Keep in mind that health risks associated with oral contraceptives go up significantly after the age of 35, especially if you're a smoker. It's important to consult with your doctor before taking oral contraceptives for acne, especially if you or any other family members have a history of blood clots. Also be sure to report any breakthrough bleeding to your doctor.

Spironolactone. This medication has been around for more than 30 years and was originally used to treat kidney problems and high blood pressure, but it's quite effective for treating acne, too. In low doses (which is what's prescribed for acne), it mainly inhibits testosterone, a "male" hormone that's also present in women.

Doctors sometimes prescribe spironolactone for women who have polycystic ovary syndrome. This disease can lead to elevated levels of "male" hormones in the blood, ovaries that don't produce eggs regularly, increased facial and body hair, and acne. Spironolactone helps reduce hair growth and control acne, and for many women, it also helps reduce PMS-type symptoms.

You shouldn't take spironolactone if you have low blood pressure, for it may lower your blood pressure just enough to make you dizzy. (This won't happen for women with normal or slightly elevated blood pressure—for them, lower blood pressure is a positive side effect.) This medication can't be taken if you're pregnant or thinking about getting pregnant, since it may affect the development of the male fetus's genitalia.

Accutane. Accutane (the brand name for isotretinoin) should be reserved for severe acne—that is, cystic or scarring acne. It's sometimes used to treat people who have tried several other acne therapies for a reasonable period of time but haven't responded.

For severe acne, especially in the teens and 20s, Accutane is far and away the most effective treatment there is. People in this category have about an 80-percent chance of not needing further oral medication after completing a six-month course of Accutane. The other 20 percent who take Accutane may have a recurrence of severe acne, in which case a second treatment can be effective. Accutane is rarely used more than twice.

Accutane should be prescribed by a board-certified dermatologist and monitored monthly or more often, and patients using it must thoroughly understand the side effects of this drug. Prevention of pregnancy with two methods of birth control (for example, oral contraceptives plus condoms) is a must, since the drug can cause severe birth defects if taken during pregnancy.

Your dermatologist will require an office visit and a careful history and examination. You'll also need two negative pregnancy tests before starting Accutane, a screen of blood-fat levels (cholesterol and triglycerides), and a liver-function test.

"Is Accutane safe? I got scared to death after I read all the information on it."

Accutane has been used to help tens of thousands of people who suffer from severe acne. It's a very safe drug—when used correctly and responsibly.

Just about everyone who takes it will feel somewhat dehydrated and have dry lips, so your dermatologist will change your skin care (I often have my patients wash and moisturize with Cetaphil products for the duration of the treatment). You'll also need to use lip balm approximately once an hour to prevent them from cracking.

A monthly blood test will be done to check for pregnancy (see above). The test will include a liver test (rarely a problem unless excessive alcohol is being used) and a test for blood-fat levels, cholesterol, and triglycerides (these go up on Accutane but come back down after you've stopped taking it). I also tell my patients to report unusually severe headaches or headaches that last overnight—if you get one, don't take any more Accutane and give your doctor a call. Also, let your doctor know if you start to feel blue or depressed while you're on it (another rare side effect).

Why Accutane Is So Strictly Regulated

Accutane is a close relative of vitamin A. Too much vitamin A can cause birth defects, which is why your doctor will ask you to not take extra amounts during pregnancy. Because of this risk, your dermatologist will require you to use two methods of birth control and to take monthly pregnancy tests. But it's up to you to use that birth control and make responsible decisions regarding your sexual activity. If you've had unprotected sex while on Accutane, it's important to call your doctor and consider stopping the medication temporarily. Fortunately, Accutane is cleared out of your system fairly quickly—even so, I ask my patients who have completed a course of Accutane to wait one or two months before they try to get pregnant.

Microdermabrasion

"Will microdermabrasion help my acne?"

It depends on what type you have. If you have grade-I or grade-II acne, it should respond well after a series of treatments followed by maintenance. But other types of acne, particularly those that are inflamed, very pustular, or cystic, will get worse.

Microdermabrasion isn't advised without first seeing a dermatologist, as you may need to have the inflammation brought under control first. Many dermatologists now offer microdermabrasion in their offices so that you can be assured of getting treatment geared to your particular skin problems. In addition, experienced aestheticians may also offer this treatment.

Facials

"Are facials helpful for acne?"

Facials performed by an experienced aesthetician may be helpful if you have mild to moderate acne. The aesthetician will normally steam your face and *gently*—that's the key word—extract some of the plugs in your pores. If you bruise afterwards, find another aesthetician.

Facials can be done monthly and are usually compatible with treatments prescribed by your dermatologist. Just be sure to let the aesthetician know what medications and skin-care products you're using. If you have moderate to severe acne, find an aesthetician who works in an office with a dermatologist before undertaking any facials or microdermabrasion—if these aren't done correctly, they may make your acne worse.

SUMMARY OF ACNE: WHAT TO DO

For mild acne, you can try over-the-counter medications, which may be enough to help you. For moderate acne, see your primary-care physician or dermatologist, who can customize your treatment based on your skin type, age, and hormone activity.

If you have severe acne, see a dermatologist, who can help you prevent scarring and clear up your skin.

☙ ☙ ☙   ☙ ☙ ☙

$$\sim\!\!\diamond\!\!\sim 15 \sim\!\!\diamond\!\!\sim$$

LIVING WITH ROSACEA

Between the ages of 30 and 50, millions of people start to notice an increasing redness across their faces that doesn't go away. This condition is called *rosacea* or *adult-onset acne,* and it can look similar to the redness, bumps, and swelling of teenage acne. Regardless of what it's called, rosacea sufferers are often embarrassed by the redness—and many of them are even unfairly labeled as alcoholics because of it.

This chapter will fill you in on the basics of rosacea, including what it is, what triggers it, and how to treat it.

WHAT YOU NEED TO KNOW

- What is rosacea?
- What triggers it?

WHAT ARE THE POSSIBLE TREATMENTS?

- Lifestyle changes
- Cleansers
- Nonprescription remedies
- Prescription creams
- Oral antibiotics
- Accutane
- Lasers

WHAT YOU NEED TO KNOW

What Is Rosacea?

"My doctor tells me I have rosacea. What is this exactly?"

Rosacea is a condition that often begins as a tendency to flush or blush easily, and it gradually progresses to persistent redness and occasional swelling across the bridge of the nose and into the cheeks, forehead, and chin. As rosacea progresses, small blood vessels, red bumps, pimples, and sometimes even larger cysts appear, but unlike acne, there are no blackheads. In more advanced cases, a condition called *rhinophyma* may develop, in which thick bumps arise on the nose that may require surgery. This occurs when the oil glands and blood vessels on the nose enlarge so much that it becomes very bulbous in appearance.

Those most likely to develop rosacea are of English or Irish ancestry, but even if you don't have such genes, it may still surface. Most rosacea sufferers are fair skinned, and they tend to be women between the ages of 30 and 50—although it can occasionally affect men, teens, and menopausal women as well. Researchers don't know why women get rosacea more often than men.

Initially, the redness of rosacea may come and go, and you may not even realize that you need treatment. Keep in mind that about half of rosacea sufferers have eye symptoms, too—many experience some burning and grittiness of the eye (conjunctivitis) or inflammation and swelling of the eyelid areas. Rosacea usually becomes worse without treatment and seldom goes away on its own. So, if your skin doesn't return to its normal color, and enlarged blood vessels and pimples appear, you should see a dermatologist. The key to successful management of rosacea is early diagnosis and treatment.

What Triggers It?

"I've heard of triggers for rosacea. Can I lessen my redness without medical treatment?"

Rosacea can be set off by a number of factors, and many patients can reduce their redness by doing some detective work to figure out their own triggers. The most common are alcohol (especially red wine, beer, bourbon, gin, vodka, or champagne) and heat (saunas or hot tubs). Other people have found that the sun, strong winds, exercise, coffee or other hot drinks, certain foods (liver, dairy products, chocolate, soy products, vegetables—especially eggplant, tomatoes, and beans; fruits—including avocados, bananas, and citrus fruits; spicy foods), skin-care products (particularly sprays containing alcohol, fragrances, or witch hazel), and overuse of prescription steroid creams can stimulate their redness. In other words, triggers are very individual.

Taking the time to figure out your personal triggers will pay off in the long run. Rosacea is a disease that often starts in midlife and can continue for 10 or 20 years, so the little things that you do every day really do make a difference in the progression and treatment of this problem. The following list of suggestions should help you manage your triggers.

Avoid alcohol. Some patients with rosacea find that they tolerate white wine or certain spirits easily, but that red wine, bourbon, gin, or vodka gives them a flushed look. If you enjoy an occasional drink, you might want to experiment with different types of alcohol. For some people, the sulfites used to preserve wine are the problem rather than the wine itself—if that's the case for you, try a sulfite-free wine. And keep in mind that inexpensive wines have more additives in general.

Remember that drinking too much alcohol can cause many problems outside of causing your rosacea to flare up. For example, alcohol raises estrogens circulating in the blood, which may increase a woman's risk of breast cancer; women (for reasons that aren't entirely understood) are also more susceptible to liver damage from alcohol then men. In addition, alcohol contributes to osteoporosis.

Exercise. Exercise in a cool environment and try not to become overheated.

Pay attention to what you eat and drink. Food triggers are very

individual, so you might want to keep a food diary for several weeks to see if any foods aggravate your redness.

You also may want to try avoiding hot drinks and caffeine. Keep a log for a few weeks to see if your flushing is associated with certain drinks. If there's no association, great—there's no need to stop that beverage. But if there *is* a beverage that's causing problems, try to find a substitute for it.

Be aware of weather changes. Practice sun protection and avoid the extremes of hot and cold temperatures that tend to aggravate rosacea symptoms. Limit exposure to sunlight, wear a hat, and use broad-spectrum sunscreens with an SPF of 15 or higher.

Be gentle to your face. Avoid rubbing, scrubbing, or massaging the face, as such actions tend to irritate reddened skin.

Use nonirritating skin- and hair-care products. Try to avoid any type of hair-spray product—use gels or pomades instead. Avoid irritating cosmetics and facial products, such as Retin-A (tretinoin) or creams with high percentages of alpha-hydroxy acids.

Balance your emotions. Stress and anxiety have been reported to aggravate rosacea in some people. There are many good stress-reduction programs and gentle forms of exercise that may be beneficial for this condition, such as yoga or Pilates—just don't do them in a hot room.

———— ◈ ————

Do I Have Rosacea If I Flush and Blush Easily?

Almost everyone who gets rosacea has a history of flushing and blushing. But just because you flush, that doesn't necessarily mean that you have rosacea. Many of us flush and blush with exercise, heat, and stressful situations—the difference with early rosacea is that you might start to flush more and more frequently and with more triggers, and the redness won't go away as easily. If you're not sure if your flushing has become rosacea, make an appointment with your dermatologist to discuss it.

———— ◈ ————

POSSIBLE TREATMENTS

Lifestyle Changes

"What lifestyle changes will help my redness?"

The suggestions listed below have been known to help people with rosacea and flushing and blushing. Try them one at a time for several weeks. Redness will often wax and wane over a period of weeks or months—if you try something for just a couple of days, you really can't be sure that the change has made a difference or not. Try the following, but keep in mind that not all of these will work for everyone:

- Avoid alcohol completely or try different types (for instance, drink white wine instead of red).
- If you live in a warm climate, exercise when it's 70 degrees or cooler.
- Avoid spicy foods, coffee and caffeinated teas, and hot liquids.

- If sun seems to activate your redness, try using zinc-based sunscreen, and stay out of the sun.
- If you think you might be perimenopausal or menopausal, check with your doctor to see if estrogen replacement is advisable for other reasons as well.
- If you're pregnant, avoid getting overheated or overly fatigued.
- If you're on hormone replacement therapy (HRT), try taking your estrogen at night instead of in the morning.

"My dermatologist told me that I need to cut down on alcohol and coffee consumption and stay out of the sun if I want my rosacea to get better. Is this true?"

Lifestyle changes really are one of the mainstays of rosacea treatment. The more you eliminate the things that trigger flushing, blushing, and rosacea breakouts, the more successful your dermatologist will be with her prescription treatments.

If your rosacea is affected by your occupation, working closely with your dermatologist is even more important. Consider the case of the chef with severe rosacea: Her job requires her to work in an overheated kitchen and attend frequent wine tastings. Her rosacea can still be brought under control, but it's going to take more work.

Also, if you're a woman in your mid-40s to mid-50s, and you're having early symptoms of menopause, please consult your dermatologist. Menopausal hot flashes can aggravate rosacea and make it more difficult to control.

Cleansers

"I have rosacea. What should I be using to cleanse my skin?"

It's very important that you use nonirritating cleansers, such as Dove for sensitive skin or Cetaphil Gentle Skin Cleanser. Your dermatologist may carry nonirritating, nondrying cleansers for patients with rosacea or other skin conditions. Plexion, a prescription cleanser that contains sulfacetamide and sulfur, may be helpful as well.

Wash your face twice a day with warm water and gently pat it dry. *Do not use hot water,* as this will aggravate your redness. Next, apply your rosacea medication, followed by a gentle, nonirritating moisturizer (and don't forget your sunscreen!).

When you shower, be sure that you don't aim the spray of your high-pressure showerhead at your face, as this will make your skin very red. You should also avoid scrubs, as they're too harsh for skin with active rosacea. And your skin may not tolerate vitamin-A derivatives (such as Retin-A, most alpha-hydroxy acids, or vitamin-C lotions or creams) unless they're specifically formulated for sensitive skin.

Nonprescription Treatments

"Are there any nonprescription medicines I can use for redness?"

The only one that helps reduce redness is hydrocortisone, a very mild anti-inflammatory steroid cream that comes in either .5-percent or 1-percent strength. Even though hydrocortisone does temporarily reduce redness somewhat, it really doesn't address the root causes of rosacea at all. And it isn't nearly as effective as prescription treatments.

Using a little hydrocortisone cream while you're waiting to get in to see your doctor is probably fine, but don't use it over long periods of time or in lieu of the better prescription treatments that are available. If used incorrectly, some steroid creams can thin the skin and cause permanent dilation of its blood vessels—hydrocortisone .5-percent and 1-percent aren't strong enough to do that unless you use them many times a day over a long period of time. Be sure that you don't use them around the eye area under any circumstances without discussing it with your dermatologist first.

Prescription Creams

"I'm confused about all the different prescription creams available to treat rosacea. Can you help?"

Metronidazole has been a staple for treatment of rosacea for many years and is available in three forms: a cream, a lotion, and a gel— known respectively as MetroCream, MetroLotion, and MetroGel. These are generally prescribed for use twice a day, although if your rosacea has been stable and inactive for several months, cutting down to once a day might be fine. A relatively new cream called *Noritate* is a metronidazole cream in a different strength and is used once a day. Another common prescription for rosacea is sulfacetamide cream, and your doctor may prescribe others according to her preference.

Topical medicines are excellent at helping control rosacea and prevent recurrences, particularly over the long haul. Unfortunately, you may be disappointed if you expect them to get rid of all of your redness, particularly if you've had it for a long time, you're quite red, or you have permanently dilated small blood vessels. If you have any of those symptoms, you'll probably need laser treatments as well.

"Does it make any difference if my rosacea medication is a gel, lotion, or cream?"

All of the aforementioned preparations contain metronidazole and are equally effective—which one you should use will depend more on your underlying skin type than the fact that you have rosacea.

If you have oily or acne-prone skin, you'll probably prefer MetroGel (many male patients seem to prefer it, too). If your skin is normal or combination, then the lotion will probably be most compatible. If you're dry or over 40 years of age, MetroCream or Noritate cream would be a good choice for you.

Oral Antibiotics

"My dermatologist prescribed me MetroCream and an oral antibiotic for my rosacea. Why do I need both?"

She may have decided on this because oral antibiotics help decrease rosacea's acnelike pustules and pimples and the inflammation that can cause swelling and redness.

A common treatment approach with new active rosacea is to start metronidizole cream twice a day, in addition to an oral antibiotic for 60 days. It takes the creams about eight to ten weeks to really work, while the oral antibiotics take effect faster and then may be stopped once the cream has started to work. However, do not discontinue your oral antibiotic without discussing it with your dermatologist first. You may have the type of rosacea that needs an oral antibiotic to keep it in control. Tetracycline, doxycycline, and minocycline are prescribed most commonly, but other antibiotics may be used as well.

You should begin to see some progress in one to three weeks, with continued improvement slowly over several months. Antibiotics in the tetracycline family shouldn't be taken by pregnant women or by those actively trying to get pregnant. They can also cause increased sensitivity to the sun, so ask your doctor about continuing their use if you plan to go on vacation in a sunny place.

Amoxicillin is an alternative for a pregnant woman (or one who's trying to get pregnant) who develops rosacea. It's safe and has been used for many years (but it can't be used by anyone who's allergic to penicillin). Check with your obstetrician first.

Since medicated creams and lotions may not control rosacea 100 percent of the time, it's often wise to keep an oral antibiotic on hand in case of a sudden flare-up. These seem to be most common around the holidays when perhaps more alcohol is consumed, dietary patterns are interrupted, or stress levels increase. Other frequent times for flare-ups seems to be vacations, so be sure you take your medication with you. If you catch the flare-up early, a week or two on the antibiotic will probably suffice.

Accutane

"My sister was prescribed Accutane for her acne. Might this help my rosacea?"

Acne and rosacea are two very different diseases. Accutane should be reserved for patients who have severe cystic scarring acne or who have moderately severe acne that hasn't responded to reasonable trials of other types of therapy. Rosacea is a completely different story: It's rarely cystic and rarely scars. Accutane does, however, work well in that occasional situation where rosacea has become cystic and isn't responding to other treatment.

Accutane is a potent medication with many side effects. If you're preg-nant, are thinking about becoming pregnant, or aren't actively preventing pregnancy with birth control, you should never be using this drug, as it can cause birth defects. Always consult a doctor on the benefits and side effects of Accutane.

Lasers

"My rosacea is under control with prescription medications, but I still seem to be red. Why isn't this going away?"

Keep in mind that rosacea is only one cause of redness, so even if it's being treated, the baseline redness and dilated blood vessels may not go away with prescription medications alone. But it's important to keep using medication to keep your rosacea under control and prevent further progression of the disease.

In your situation, the best way to remove redness and dilated blood vessels and bring your skin back to its baseline color is with the gentle lasers that are now available. However, you shouldn't do this until your rosacea has been treated for at least two to four months.

It's also important to know that after you've finished your laser treatments, you'll probably need periodic maintenance treatments to maintain your baseline color. The more you flush and blush or do other things that aggravate redness, such as drinking wine or spending time in the heat or sun, the more often you'll need these maintenance treatments. Ask your dermatologist for a reasonable estimate of what you can expect.

When Should I Consider Getting Laser Treatments?

Since being red doesn't hurt you, the answer could be "never." Laser treatments for redness or dilated blood vessels are really a cosmetic issue, but it might be time to consider them in the following instances:

1. Your flushing is bad enough that it's interfering with your work or social life (for example, if you're avoiding speaking in public because you're afraid you might flush or blush).

2. You've had people assume that you're a heavy drinker because your nose and cheeks are red. (You can also try just educating your friends and co-workers about rosacea.)

3. You're having to pile on the makeup in the morning just to feel presentable.

4. You have a strong family history of rosacea, and you know your condition is probably going to worsen over the next several years.

SUMMARY OF ROSACEA: WHAT TO DO

Rosacea is a disease that often gets worse if you don't do anything about it. To prevent its progression, see your dermatologist for advice on your particular situation.

In general, you should be able to get your rosacea under control if you:

•   apply gentle cleansers, sunscreens, and moisturizers;

•   adopt a lifestyle that minimizes your own triggers for rosacea; and

•   use prescription creams or antibiotics.

Once your rosacea is treated and under control, you may want to consider getting gentle laser treatments to reduce the remaining redness and/or dilated blood vessels.

❖ 16 ❖

SENSITIVE SKIN, SKIN ALLERGIES, AND ECZEMA

Sensitive skin seems to flare up at the mildest provocation: A piece of jewelry, a skin product, or even exposure to light can set it off. Allergy testing is often the best way to get to the bottom of why your skin is sensitive, and medications can be very helpful in reducing allergic reactions. In addition, lifestyle changes, as well as avoiding the substance you're allergic to, will give you the best chance of keeping your skin clear and healthy.

This chapter will provide you with the basics on sensitive skin and skin allergies. It also covers eczema, because this affliction goes hand-in-hand with many skin allergies.

SKIN-SENSITIVITY ISSUES

- What is sensitive skin?
- Eczema
- Lip problems
- Environmental irritants
- Allergy testing

WHAT ARE THE POSSIBLE TREATMENTS?

- Lifestyle changes
- Nonprescription remedies
- Prescription medications
- Therapeutic light treatments

SKIN-SENSITIVITY ISSUES

What Is Sensitive Skin?

"I seem to have a lot of problems with skin-care products. Does this mean I have sensitive skin?"

Yes. Having sensitive skin usually just means that it gets irritated easily. The cause can be something as simple as exfoliating too much with scrubs and loofah sponges, for abrasive cleaners can certainly make the skin irritated and red. Also, your skin just may not tolerate some products, such as vitamin-A derivatives (like Retin-A), alpha-hydroxy acids, or those products that have an acid pH. But these are irritant reactions, not true allergies.

True skin allergies are often caused by products containing perfume, lanolin, or preservatives—or even to the metal in jewelry. Many people with sensitive skin do have atopic dermatitis (eczema), yet they may not necessarily have a family history of allergies, asthma, eczema, or hay fever. Your dermatologist can help you sort this out.

"I'm 16, and everyone in my family seems to have sensitive skin, eczema, or other problems with their skin. Am I going to have these problems, too?"

It's quite likely—problems with skin run in families for the simple reason that our genes carry certain skin diseases with them. Four diseases—eczema, allergies, asthma, and hay fever—are coded together on the same gene complex, which is sometimes referred to as an *atopic gene.* The eczema associated with this gene is called *atopic eczema* or *atopic dermatitis.* Atopic eczema is very common in all parts of the world, affecting about 10 percent of babies and about 3 percent of the overall population in the United States.

Your family tree may show eczema and allergies in some members of the family and hay fever and asthma in others—some unlucky individuals will probably even inherit all four of those problems. If you have them on just one side of your family, you're better off than if such afflictions run on both sides. And while most people with atopic eczema have family members with similar problems, as many as 20 percent of eczema sufferers may be the only ones in their family who have it.

Eczema

"I'm in my early 20s. I had eczema as a baby, and now I seem to be developing problems again. Is this unusual?"

Almost half of all babies with eczema will grow out of it; the other half will have some degree of eczema (also called *dermatitis*) throughout their lives. And it's not unusual for this type of eczema to go away for a period of time and then recur.

In early childhood, eczema is often very red, blistering, and crusty. In the adult form, lesions tend to be drier and reddish brown, while the skin itself is scaly and thickened. Both children and adults tend to find the red, scaly patches to be unbearably itchy, particularly at night—some patients scratch them in their sleep until they bleed.

If your eczema is mild, first try the measures suggested in this chapter on lifestyle changes. If it's more severe, you'll need to see a good dermatologist.

"I have fairly severe eczema that affects my face. Could allergies to my skin-care products be causing this problem?"

It's important to see your dermatologist to get an accurate diagnosis, because there are many different types of eczema.

If you have dry, itchy skin with a rash, along with a personal or family history of allergies, asthma, or hay fever, you may have atopic eczema. You could also have a specific allergy to one or more ingredients commonly found in skin- and hair-care products and nail polish. Or you could have both—that is, you may have atopic eczema *and* an allergy to various ingredients in skin-care products. Your dermatologist may suggest allergy testing to figure out what's causing your reactions.

Dermatologists test for allergens likely to cause skin problems, such as nickel (in jewelry), formaldehyde-releasing agents (common preservatives used in all sorts of creams), fragrances, and so forth. Allergists usually test for reactions to foods (such as cow's milk, soy, eggs, fish, wheat, peanuts, citrus fruits, nuts, tomatoes, and products containing gluten) or things in the environment

(such as dust mites, pollens, or grasses). Allergists usually test for reactions to foods (such as cow's milk, soy, eggs, fish, wheat, peanuts, citrus fruits, nuts, tomatoes, and products containing gluten) or things in the environment (such as dust mites, pollens, or grasses).

Lip Problems

"My lips are always chapped, even when the weather is warm. Why does this happen?"

You may lick your lips a lot, which tends to dry them out and leads to chapping. Try breaking this habit by using lip balm ten to twenty times a day instead—once you've stopped licking, you can cut back to three or four times.

You could also be allergic to an ingredient in your lip balm, toothpaste, or lipstick. Red lipstick in particular can contain dyes that cause allergic reactions—try choosing a sheer color instead. And although cinnamon-flavored lip balms may smell or taste good, they have a higher chance of causing allergic reactions on the lips.

If you eat a lot of fruit, you may be reacting to the acid in the juice or have an allergy to that particular fruit. If you think this might be the case, try cutting the fruit into small pieces so that it doesn't touch your lips.

To keep your lips smooth, use a balm that has sunscreen, natural oils, or petroleum in it. L'Occitane makes one that's pure shea butter (a nut oil), which you can layer over a sunscreen. Keep the balm by your bed so that you can reapply it if you wake up during the night. You could also try applying a thin layer of one-percent hydrocortisone ointment to your lips before bedtime to soothe the irritation for one to two weeks. And avoid aggravating the chapping by licking, picking at, or biting your lips.

"I often have sores at the corners of my mouth. What causes this?"

The same principles with chapped lips apply here but with a couple of differences. Since the corners of the mouth retain moisture, they can become infected with yeast or bacteria (usually staph). If you don't improve with the measures listed above, try eliminating fluoride and flavorings except mint in your toothpaste. Try Lotrimin cream (an anti-yeast medication), three times a day for one to two weeks. If you're still not better, your dermatologist can do a culture to see if bacteria are the problem or if you need allergy testing.

Dos and Don'ts for Lips

- Do use sunscreen on your lips several times a day, as lips are one of the most common sites for non-melanoma skin cancers.
- Do apply lipstick over your sunscreen, or wear lip balms and lipstick with sunscreen already in it. Try Bobbi Brown Essentials.
- Don't lick your lips. The constant wetting and drying takes off your sunscreen and causes chapping.
- Do apply a lip balm at night. Try L'Occitane shea butter balm or SkinCeuticals antioxidant lip repair.

Environmental Irritants

"I have severe eczema and lots of problems with my skin. Could environmental agents be aggravating this condition?"

It's difficult to know, because so many things that we're exposed to on a daily basis can irritate us, including climate changes, various foods and the chemicals in them, detergents and cleansers, fabric softeners, aerosolized or airborne allergens, and coatings on virtually every item we use. Even plain old dust can be to blame—dust mites and dust-catching objects such as feather pillows, down comforters, mattresses, carpeting, drapes, toys, and rough fabrics such as wool may cause atopic dermatitis to worsen.

In addition, very dry environments will aggravate eczema. Often eczema will get worse in the fall in cold climates when the central heating goes on—or in the summer in hot areas where air conditioning is used quite a bit.

It can be almost impossible to isolate what's causing a particular individual's problem, but your dermatologist and allergist will do their best through a series of tests (explained later in the chapter).

"I seem to develop a rash whenever I use perfume. Is there anything I can do about this?"

Fragrances are one of the most common causes of allergic skin rashes, as they're lurking in many skin-care products and cosmetics. If you're sensitive to fragrances, it's best to avoid them in all of your skin-care products. But if the problem is mild, you might try using perfume on your clothing instead of directly on your skin. Or you may be able to use perfume from a bottle but not a spray, since sprays contain agents that aerosolize chemicals, which can cause irritation. In addition, make sure that you don't put perfume on the sides of your neck during the day, as many fragrances interact with sunlight to create a blotchy appearance, which can sometimes become permanent.

Almost all of the skin-care lines found in dermatologists' offices are fragrance free, as are some at department stores and drugstores. Look at the Clinique, Prescriptives, Cetaphil, and Eucerin lines.

If you have problems with lipstick or colored blush and eye shadows, you may be reacting to a specific dye. Experiment with different shades of red or a more brown or pink tone to see if that makes a difference. You should test cosmetics on your inner forearm to make sure you don't have a reaction before you apply them to your face.

"I get a rash on my ears every time I wear a certain pair of earrings. What's causing this?"

Skin is often irritated by certain alloys in metals (usually cheap ones), most commonly nickel and cobalt. Such allergies may be very mild or they may be extremely severe. In fact, some people are so sensitive to nickel that even the small amounts in coins, doorknobs, and the metal handles of kitchen instruments may cause a reaction.

Nickel can lurk in unsuspecting places, such as watches, eyeglasses, bra clasps, and grommets used in pants. If your skin develops a rash in an area where it's contacting one of the above, that's a big clue that you have a nickel allergy.

Kits are available to test metals quickly and easily for nickel content. Your dermatologist can do a patch test for nickel and cobalt allergies and can also suggest ways to protect your hands from metals.

Allergy Testing

"I have moderately severe eczema, and my dermatologist suggested allergy testing. Why?"

One of the most effective ways to treat eczema is to eliminate the things that may be aggravating it. An allergy test may identify what worsens your eczema so that you can then avoid that substance.

If you have eczema, you may also have allergies, asthma, or hay fever, so it makes sense to do some formal testing for these problems. You can be tested for allergies to dust, pollen, animal hair, and many other common irritants.

You'll need to see an allergist, who will inject a tiny amount of an extract of the irritant under your skin with a very small needle. (The needle is so tiny that the injection is usually hardly felt.) The allergist will then look for a certain type of reaction to the skin and will grade it according to its severity. She'll also give you advice on what to avoid and how to do it. The latter part is critical, because some allergens are very common, and decreasing your exposure to them can be difficult. Allergy shots may also be suggested depending on the problem.

Although instituting the measures that your allergist suggests probably won't cure your eczema, it could make it less severe; her suggestions can also enhance the success of the medications and lifestyle changes your dermatologist recommends.

"My dermatologist suggests that we do patch testing. Can you explain what this is?"

Patch testing checks for a completely different set of substances than allergy tests. Allergists test for things such as grass, pollen, mold, dust mites, and food. But dermatologists use patch testing to test skin for allergies to items such as latex, lanolin, preservatives, fragrances, ingredients in skin-care products, and the like.

In a patch test, your doctor will tape small discs or patches with tiny amounts of various substances to your skin. A waterproof covering can be placed over the patches so you can shower, but you'll be asked not to swim or exercise vigorously, as too much water or sweat will dislodge the patches.

The discs are read at different intervals by your doctor, usually 48 or 72 hours, and possibly again at about 96 hours. If you develop a red spot under the patch, then the test is positive—you have an allergy to that substance. Your dermatologist may also want to check the sites one week later for any late reactions.

How does your doctor know which substance to check for an allergic reaction? The most common test uses two small strips containing the 24 substances that are statistically the most likely to cause or aggravate eczema, but there are hundreds of other substances that can cause allergic reactions. In most large cities, there are at least one or two dermatologists who specialize in this type of testing and have hundreds of allergens available to use should the standard 24 be negative. Your dermatologist may refer you to one of these patch-testing experts if she doesn't specialize in this area herself. Also, your dermatologist may suggest what's sometimes called a *use test*, where a small amount of a product such as hair spray, shampoo, or even shoe leather is put under a patch and left on the forearm or another site for several days.

You should stop taking all antihistamines for at least three to seven days prior to patch testing, because they can skew the result. Also, if your eczema is severe, your dermatologist may wait to test you until it's under better control. You may also be asked to wait if you're taking prednisone.

෨ ෨ ෨

POSSIBLE TREATMENTS

Lifestyle Changes

"My doctor gave me a whole list of things to change in my life. Do I really need to do all of them?"

Yes. It would be so nice if there were a magic pill for eczema, but there isn't. Treating it successfully often just comes down to hard work and attention to detail. But once new habits are instituted, life gets easier and your skin will improve immensely.

Here are some of the main lifestyle changes you can implement to improve your eczema or sensitive skin:

- Take only short lukewarm showers or baths. Hot water increases itching in the long run, even though it may feel good initially. And staying in baths or showers for a long time actually dries your skin out and makes it itchier.

- Use only mild cleansers that don't strip oil off your skin. Try Dove products for sensitive skin or Cetaphil Gentle Skin Cleanser.

- Use cleansers only on your face, armpits, and groin. Unless you've been mountain biking or doing something really dirty, there's no need to use cleansers on your entire body.

- Use a high-quality hypoallergenic lotion once or twice a day all over your body, particularly on your arms and legs. It's very important that you do this daily. Good suggestions are Cetaphil cream or lotion, Eucerin cream or lotion, Vanicream, or even just plain old Vaseline.

- Use a hypoallergenic detergent such as All-free, Tide-free, or Cheer-free. *Do not* use any fabric softeners—even the ones that say "hypoallergenic" can leave tiny, irritating fibers all over your clothes. Don't overload the washer, and try using a double-rinse cycle.

- Avoid perfumes, scented aftershave lotions or sprays, and spray products such as hair spray or cleaning products. These aerosolized chemicals can aggravate eczema.

- If you exercise regularly, try to rinse the sweat off as soon as possible, and apply more lotion.

- If you have a rash on your face or neck, your shampoo or conditioner may be contributing to the problem. Try Free and Clear (in the Vanicream line) shampoo and conditioner, which is formulated for people who have sensitive skin or eczema.

- Try to wear cotton clothing and avoid wool if it's itchy.

- Consider using a humidifier at home (particularly in the bedroom) to increase the moisture content in the air. And remove environmental allergens, such as dust and pet hair, from your home.

- With moderate or severe eczema (as with many diseases), you should always try to get plenty of sleep, eat a healthy balanced diet, and try to reduce stress.

If you've had allergy testing or patch testing, then your doctors may have asked you to avoid or change other things depending on the results of those tests. You should follow those instructions to the letter.

Nonprescription Remedies

"I have dry, itchy skin with occasional patches of eczema. Is there anything I can use from the drugstore, or do I have to go see my doctor?"

If your eczema is mild, you can definitely try taking nonprescription remedies first. If, by the end of a week or two, your eczema isn't gone or it's become severe, you need to make an appointment with your dermatologist.

The first thing to do is to try all of the measures listed above. Get a mild, nonirritating cleanser such as Cetaphil, and use a high-quality hypoallergenic moisturizer such as Vanicream or Cetaphil cream once or twice a day all over. One-percent hydrocortisone cream or ointment may also be useful: Apply it several times a day for the first few days and then once a day for a week or two if needed. In general, ointments are better for eczema than creams because they hold water in the skin better and contain fewer ingredients that might irritate you. However, it isn't always feasible to use ointment on your face because it leaves a shiny, greasy film. Keep in mind that you may become allergic to hydrocortisone over time, so if your

eczema to be getting worse when you use it, stop right away and call your doctor.

If the eczema is on your face and you have acne, the measures above may aggravate the acne. You should definitely seek medical advice.

The eye area. The eyelids are one of the most common places for eczema problems. The culprit here is usually eye makeup. If this is true for you, first try paring down to these three products—mascara, a basic liner, and a concealer. Buy those three products in a line that tends to be more hypoallergenic, such as Almay (sold in drugstores) or Clinique (found in department stores). The concealer can be used on dark circles or can be worn on the lids if you're used to wearing eye shadow. If your eczema clears up, don't just start using your regular products all at once—add them back in one at a time about four or five days apart so that you can identify the offending agent easily if you flare up again. If that doesn't work, stop everything and see your dermatologist.

Also, keep in mind that problems on the eyelids are often caused by minute amounts of substances transferred from your hands to your eyes. This is particularly true with nail polish. Don't touch or rub the eye area for at least three or four hours after applying polish. And it's best not to touch or rub your eyes at all unless you've washed them with a hypoallergenic cleanser and rinsed well.

Infections. Most eczema will itch slightly, but it's usually not sore. So if you have tenderness or pain, swelling, increased warmth or heat, a break in the skin, pus, yellow crusts, or your eczema seems to be spreading rapidly, you may have an infection. For instance, impetigo (an infection on the face caused by a bacteria called *staph* or *strep*) may often look like eczema in adults.

Call your dermatologist right away. She may want to do a culture to identify the bacteria, and you'll probably need antibiotics. An antibiotic cream called *Bactroban* (mupirocin) may be used instead of oral antibiotics in some situations. Also, you may be asked to apply an antibiotic cream inside your nostrils for a while, because the bacteria will sometimes live up there in what's called the *carrier state*.

Prescription Medications

"Over the years, my dermatologists have given me a number of different creams. What's the difference between them?"

This may be a confusing area because there are literally dozens of different options for treating eczema. Often the same medication with a long name will come in an ointment, cream, lotion, and solution depending on the problem and the part of the body it's prescribed for. To make matters worse, the medications often come in several different strengths, which can make quite a difference in how it affects you.

Please keep in mind that none of your medications will be very effective without the lifestyle changes mentioned earlier in this chapter. Those are just as important as your medications in keeping your eczema under control in the long run.

Let's look at the primary medications used to treat eczema and atopic dermatitis.

Topical steroids. These are in a completely different class from the kinds of steroids that body builders or weight lifters use. When prescribed by a dermatologist in the right strength for the right period of time, these medications are extremely safe and effectively relieve itching and redness.

Topical steroids are generally lumped into low potency, mid potency, and high potency. High-potency topical steroids should never be used continually for long without a dermatologist's directions, nor should they be used on the face or in the groin area. Those used on the face are usually low to mid potency and are often formulated especially for that area, so no thinning of the skin or broken blood vessels will occur.

Antihistamines. These are frequently used and are very helpful for reducing the intense itching that often accompanies eczema, and can disrupt your sleep. Scratching can both aggravate eczema and transfer the bacteria that may cause infections.

Your doctor will probably prescribe an oral antihistamine. The newer ones, such as Zyrtec, Clarinex, and Allegra, are less sedating, longer acting, and are usually taken only once or twice a day. They take two to four days to be effective, so don't give up if you don't feel that your itching is better after a day or two.

Older, shorter-acting antihistamines, such as Benadryl or Hydroxyzine, may also work well and are much less expensive than the newer agents are. These are sometimes prescribed for nighttime because they do cause drowsiness, which may wear off after three or four days on the medication. It's extremely important that you don't drive at all if these medications make you drowsy, and you shouldn't combine them with alcohol.

Protopic and Elidel. These are exciting new medications that act by quieting down the cells in your skin that are causing the inflammation in the first place. Since these cells are from your own immune system, the medications are sometimes referred to as *immune system modulators*. They don't thin the skin or cause enlargement of its tiny blood vessels the way high-potency topical steroids sometimes can.

Protopic comes in two different strengths: One is better for more sensitive areas of the body such as the face or the groin, while the other is better for your arms, legs, and trunk. Protopic may be used by itself or in combination with other topical medications, and some patients find that it can replace their topical steroids.

Antibiotics. Antibiotics are often used for more severe eczema cases or if certain kinds of staph or strep bacteria are present. It's extremely important to take antibiotics if you have these bacteria, because they live in the skin, aggravate your eczema, and prevent healing. Your dermatologist may prescribe them for anywhere from a week to even a month or two if needed, but they're generally prescribed for no more than absolutely necessary and for a limited time. Your doctor may request a follow-up culture to make sure that the bacteria are gone.

Therapeutic Light Treatments

"I have severe atopic eczema and my doctor is suggesting light treatments. Can you explain these to me?"

Light has been used for centuries in the treatment of a number of skin diseases, including psoriasis and severe atopic eczema. It acts by helping to calm down the cells in the immune system that are hyperactive in the skin and causing such conditions.

There are three types of light therapy. Just plain ultraviolet-B (UVB) is the oldest form and was often used in conjunction with tar-based products. This is not done as much anymore, and such therapy has been replaced largely by PUVA therapy and narrow-band UVB—both of which can be very effective for psoriasis and severe atopic eczema.

Light treatments are done in a "light box," which looks like one of those photo booths found in amusement arcades or county fairs. The door is closed so that you have complete privacy, and you only expose the parts of your body that have eczema to the light for several seconds or minutes.

A series of light treatments lasts several months. A typical schedule might be something like three times a week for about a month, then twice a week for about a month, and then once a week for a month or two. However, there are a lot of different regimens for light treatment, and your dermatologist will customize a regimen just for you.

Prior to your light treatment, you may be asked to take a medication containing *psoralens*—this is PUVA therapy. It's very important to follow all your dermatologist's and nurse's instructions regarding psoralens, and you'll be asked to wear protective eyewear while you're taking it. If your eczema is limited to your hands and feet, they can be soaked in psoralens first and then exposed to the light without the necessity of taking the drug internally.

Narrow-band UVB may be used in place of PUVA. It's also very effective and has the advantage of not requiring the psoralens to be taken ahead of time, so no special eyewear is needed. It's given in a similar regimen, usually starting with three times a week and then tapering off over a period of months.

Light treatments are often used in conjunction with other prescription medications mentioned above, may provide quite a long remission, and are extremely helpful in some cases of severe eczema.

SUMMARY OF SENSITIVE-SKIN ISSUES: WHAT TO DO

If your problems with sensitive skin or skin allergies aren't too severe, try the lifestyle changes discussed in this chapter. Pay close attention to skin-care products that may be causing your problem and try a regimen of mild, nonirritating cleansers and moisturizers twice a day. One-percent hydrocortisone cream is also fine for a week or two.

If your eczema is severe, you need expert advice—see your dermatologist. She may recommend allergy or patch testing to get to the bottom of what's irritating your skin; she may also prescribe medications to help you. If you're willing to do the work, there's a lot that can be done now to ease the discomfort and appearance of eczema.

෨ ෨ ෨   ෨ ෨ ෨

Afterword

It's Never Too Late

Many of my patients worry that it's too late to do anything about their skin. All those years using baby oil, cocoa butter, iodine, and reflectors; those hours spent in tanning booths; and those sunny days spent on skis, boats, and mountaintops have added up. However, if I could convey one thing, it would be this: *It's never too late.* You can't take back all those hours in the sun, nor would you necessarily want to. But skin has amazing powers of regeneration and renewal. Will it be the same as when you were 16? Of course not. However, almost everyone can have better and sometimes even great skin with a little daily attention, sun sense, and some of the new tools that we now have access to.

I tell my patients that I don't expect them to live in a cave—*I* certainly don't. I have three children whom I love to go to the beach with; we take occasional vacations in very sunny places (after all, we live in rainy Seattle); and I like to run, hike, bicycle, picnic, and enjoy our occasional good weather. It's just that I do all of this with lots of sunscreen, a nice hat, and protective clothing if it's really hot or it's midday.

If you protect your skin, use the best sunscreens and renewal products such as tretinoin, hydroxy acids, and viamin C available, and slowly invest in photorejuvenation, microdermabrasion, a little Botox, or whatever makes sense for your particular face and skin, you'll see a noticeable difference in your skin over the next year. And if you keep it up over the next three to five years, you'll see a *big* difference. I know this is true because I see it in my patients all the time.

Think of this process like making the decision to exercise, stop smoking, eat more healthfully, or relax—the small daily things make a big difference over time. And taking better care of your skin requires only an extra ten minutes out of your routine. The payoff is less risk of skin cancer, fewer wrinkles, and better skin tone and color.

MY SKIN-CARE REGIMEN

I get asked so frequently what I use that I'll answer that question here. Please keep in mind that what works for me may not work for you at all. Also bear in mind that skin health and beauty result from daily skin care, sun protection, general health, genes, and other factors—one of which is sheer luck in avoiding diseases and accidents. So you'll want to have your skin care customized for you by your dermatologist.

My Morning Routine

Cleanser: M.D. Forté Facial Cleanser I
Sunscreen: SkinCeuticals Daily Defense SPF 20 or Ultimate UV
    Defense SPF 30 (summer) or Cetaphil Daily Facial Moisturizer
    SPF 15 (winter)
Eyes: Dermalogica Total Eye Care (with alpha-hydroxy acid and SPF 15)

My Evening Routine

Cleanser: Same as above
Renewal: I alternate these every third night in this order:
    Night 1: Renova .02 percent
    Night 2: Primacy C & E
    Night 3: NeoStrata Skin Smoothing Lotion (with alpha-hydroxy
        acid) or Kinerase
Moisturizer: M.D. Forté Replenish Hydrating Cream (only if I need it)
Eyes: Primacy Eye Balm by SkinCeuticals

I often try new products, but I only use them on half my face and then compare the two sides after 30 to 90 days. If I don't see any difference, I go back to the above regimen.

My regimen may seem too complicated, but there are now many good skin-care options that are simpler. **At least start with a gentle cleanser and sunscreen in the morning and the same cleanser and one renewal product at night.**

I know that if you believe your skin looks good, you'll feel more confident. I hope this extra confidence will translate into more vitality and energy, which will help you reach out to your family and community and give something positive back to the world.

☙ ☙ ☙   ☙ ☙ ☙

APPENDIX

Internet Resources

American Academy of Dermatology (AAD): www.aad.org. This comprehensive Website for consumers covers all areas of dermatology diagnosis, disease processes, the newest treatment options, and links to a variety of other dermatology Websites.

The mailing address, phone and fax of the AAD Washington office is: American Academy of Dermatology; 1350 I Street, Suite 880; Washington, DC 20005-4355; (202) 842-3555; (202) 842-4355 (fax).

DERMAdoctor.com: www.dermadoctor.com. Created by Dr. Audrey Kunin, a dermatologist, this site features articles and newsletters where Dr. Kunin shares the most current developments in skin-care technology and research; it also offers a wide variety of skin-care products and product descriptions.

Dermatologist Skin Care: www.dermatologistskincare.com. This site sells high-quality skin-care products at competitive prices, with excellent customer service. All products and information have been reviewed by a board-certified dermatologist.

***Dermatology Times:* www.dermatologytimes.com**. This magazine provides coverage of news, research, and products related to dermatology.

***Dr. Irwin's Website:* www.madisonskin.com**. If you live in the Puget Sound area, this is how you can find my office, the Madison Skin and Laser Center.

Facefacts.com: **www.facefacts.com**. A comprehensive Website for patients dealing with acne that allows readers to e-mail questions to a physician, read about up-to-date treatment options, and separate fact from fiction.

Hair Loss: **www.hairloss.com**. The Hairloss Information Center is the ultimate resource for honest facts about hair loss. Learn about the very latest developments in hair loss, hair-loss control, hair regrowth, hair replacement, male-pattern baldness, female alopecia, Propecia, Minoxidil, and Rogaine.

National Eczema Association: **www.nationaleczema.org**. The National Eczema Association for Science and Education works to improve the health and the quality of life of persons living with atopic dermatitis/eczema, including those who have the disease as well as their loved ones.

National Psoriasis Foundation: **www.psoriasis.org**. A very comprehensive site for patients dealing with psoriasis and their loved ones, it includes all the latest treatment options along with research information, news, and events, plus media resources and links.

PsoriasisNet: **www.skincarepphysicians.com/psoriasisnet**. An authoritative source of information about psoriasis. PsoriasisNet is an on-line patient education service of the American Academy of Dermatology.

Renova: **www.renova.pill-store.co.uk**. This site reports on skin-care advances, with information on skin care, wrinkles, products, options, dermatology, and more. It also has an on-line store where products can be purchased.

The Skin Cancer Foundation: **www.skincancer.org**. The Skin Cancer Foundation is the only organization concerned exclusively with the world's most common malignancy—cancer of the skin.

Skin Store: **www.skinstore.com**. Skin Store offers more than 500 products that have undergone years of testing, approval, and daily use by clinical researchers, dermatologists, and plastic surgeons. Brands such as Cetaphil, Dermablend, and M.D. Forté, to name just a few, are featured.

Warts: **www.aad.org/pamphlets/warts.html**. This is a complete pamphlet (or article) dealing with common warts, foot warts, and flat warts; causes, treatment options, and sorting fact from fiction.

ೞ ೞ ೞ   ೞ ೞ ೞ

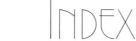

INDEX

Page numbers for sidebars are in *italics*

203

Simple index page.

NOTES

NOTES

Notes

Notes

About the Authors

Brandith Irwin practices medical and cosmetic dermatology at her own clinic, the Madison Skin and Laser Center (**www.madisonskin.com**). *Seattle* magazine recently named her one of the city's best dermatologists, based on a poll of 2,500-area doctors and nurses.

Brandith graduated with honors from the University of Washington Medical School and did residencies in both internal medicine and dermatology there. She received one of the few National Dermatology Foundation Research Fellowship Awards in 1990. Brandith is board certified in both internal medicine and dermatology and has held both full-time and clinical-faculty positions in the department of dermatology at the University of Washington.

Mark McPherson (Brandith's husband) is a writer, prize-winning poet, and lawyer with both a Ph.D. and a J.D. from Harvard.

☙ ☙ ☙

We hope you enjoyed this Hay House book.
If you would like to receive a free catalog
featuring additional Hay House books and
products, or if you would like information
about the Hay Foundation, please contact:

Hay House, Inc.
P.O. Box 5100
Carlsbad, CA 92018-5100

(760) 431-7695 or **(800) 654-5126**
(760) 431-6948 (fax) or **(800) 650-5115 (fax)**
www.hayhouse.com

☙ ☙ ☙

Published and distributed in Australia by:
Hay House Australia Pty Ltd, P.O. Box 515,
Brighton-Le-Sands, NSW 2216 • *phone:* 1800 023 516
e-mail: info@hayhouse.com.au

Distributed in the United Kingdom by:
Airlift, 8 The Arena, Mollison Ave.,
Enfield, Middlesex, United Kingdom EN3 7NL

Distributed in Canada by:
Raincoast, 9050 Shaughnessy St.,
Vancouver, B.C., Canada V6P 6E5

☙ ☙ ☙